D1033979

Pathophysiology and Care Protocols for Nursing Management

Editors

LYNN C. PARSONS
MARIA A. REVELL

NURSING CLINICS
OF NORTH AMERICA

www.nursing.theclinics.com

Consulting Editor
STEPHEN D. KRAU

December 2015 • Volume 50 • Number 4

DISCARDED

LIBRARY
FORSYTH TECHNICAL COMMUNITY COLLEGE
2100 SILAS CREEK PARKWAY
WINSTON SALEM, N.C. 27103

ELSEVIER

1600 John F. Kennedy Boulevard • Suite 1800 • Philadelphia, Pennsylvania, 19103-2899

http://www.theclinics.com

NURSING CLINICS OF NORTH AMERICA Volume 50, Number 4
December 2015 ISSN 0029-6465, ISBN-13: 978-0-323-40256-9

Editor: Kerry Holland
Developmental Editor: Casey Jackson

© **2015 Elsevier Inc. All rights reserved.**

This periodical and the individual contributions contained in it are protected under copyright by Elsevier, and the following terms and conditions apply to their use:

Photocopying
Single photocopies of single articles may be made for personal use as allowed by national copyright laws. Permission of the Publisher and payment of a fee is required for all other photocopying, including multiple or systematic copying, copying for advertising or promotional purposes, resale, and all forms of document delivery. Special rates are available for educational institutions that wish to make photocopies for non-profit educational classroom use. For information on how to seek permission visit www.elsevier.com/permissions or call: (+44) 1865 843830 (UK)/ (+1) 215 239 3804 (USA).

Derivative Works
Subscribers may reproduce tables of contents or prepare lists of articles including abstracts for internal circulation within their institutions. Permission of the Publisher is required for resale or distribution outside the institution. Permission of the Publisher is required for all other derivative works, including compilations and translations (please consult www.elsevier.com/permissions).

Electronic Storage or Usage
Permission of the Publisher is required to store or use electronically any material contained in this periodical, including any article or part of an article (please consult www.elsevier.com/permissions). Except as outlined above, no part of this publication may be reproduced, stored in a retrieval system or transmitted in any form or by any means, electronic, mechanical, photocopying, recording or otherwise, without prior written permission of the Publisher.

Notice
No responsibility is assumed by the Publisher for any injury and/or damage to persons or property as a matter of products liability, negligence or otherwise, or from any use or operation of any methods, products, instructions or ideas contained in the material herein. Because of rapid advances in the medical sciences, in particular, independent verification of diagnoses and drug dosages should be made.

Although all advertising material is expected to conform to ethical (medical) standards, inclusion in this publication does not constitute a guarantee or endorsement of the quality or value of such product or of the claims made of it by its manufacturer.

Nursing Clinics of North America (ISSN 0029-6465) is published quarterly by Elsevier Inc., 360 Park Avenue South, New York, NY 10010-1710. Months of issue are March, June, September, and December. Periodicals postage paid at New York, NY and additional mailing offices. Subscription price per year is, $150.00 (US individuals), $400.00 (US institutions), $275.00 (international individuals), $488.00 (international institutions), $220.00 (Canadian individuals), $488.00 (Canadian institutions), $85.00 (US students), and $135.00 (international students). To receive student/resident rate, orders must be accompanied by name of affiliated institution, date of term, and the signature of program/residency coordinator on institution letterhead. Orders will be billed at individual rate until proof of status is received. Foreign air speed delivery is included in all *Clinics* subscription prices. All prices are subject to change without notice. **POSTMASTER:** Send address changes to *Nursing Clinics*, Elsevier Health Sciences Division, Subscription Customer Service, 3251 Riverport Lane, Maryland Heights, MO 63043. **Customer Service: Telephone: 1-800-654-2452** (U.S. and Canada); **1-314-447-8871 (outside U.S. and Canada). Fax: 1-314-447-8029. E-mail: journalscustomerservice-usa@elsevier.com** (for print support) and **journalsonlinesupport-usa@elsevier.com** (for online support).

Nursing Clinics of North America is covered in *EMBASE/Excerpta Medica, MEDLINE/PubMed (Index Medicus), Social Sciences Citation Index, Current Contents, ASCA, Cumulative Index to Nursing, RNdex Top 100,* and Allied Health Literature and International Nursing Index (INI).

Printed in the United States of America.

Contributors

CONSULTING EDITOR

STEPHEN D. KRAU, PhD, RN, CNE
Associate Professor, Vanderbilt University Medical Center, School of Nursing, Nashville, Tennessee

EDITORS

LYNN C. PARSONS, PhD, MSN, RN, NEA-BC
Professor and Department Chair, Department of Nursing, Center for Health, Education and Research, Morehead State University, Morehead, Kentucky

MARIA A. REVELL, PhD, MSN, RN, COI
Associate Professor and MSN Program Director, Division of Nursing, Tennessee State University, School of Nursing, Nashville, Tennessee

AUTHORS

BRIANNA ABBOTT, BS
Physician Assistant Student, College of Health Science, Bethel University, McKenzie, Tennessee

NATHANIA BUSH, DNP, PHCNS-BC
Associate Professor, Department of Nursing, Morehead State University, Morehead, Kentucky

TASHA CEASS, BA
Training and Process Specialist, Medtronic, Inc., Minneapolis, Minnesota

SAMANTHA CONKLIN, MSN, FNP-BC
School of Nursing, Northern Michigan University, Marquette, Michigan

TERESA D. FERGUSON, DNP, RN, CNE
Associate Professor, Department of Nursing, Morehead State University; Staff Nurse, St. Claire Regional Medical Center, Morehead, Kentucky

LISA SUE FLOOD, DNP
Professor, School of Nursing, Northern Michigan University, Marquette, Michigan

NANCI K. GASIEWICZ, DNP, RN, CNE
Associate Dean and Director, School of Nursing, Northern Michigan University, Marquette, Michigan

TERESA L. HOWELL, DNP, RN, CNE
Professor, Department of Nursing, Morehead State University, Morehead, Kentucky

RICHARD P. LAKSONEN Jr, Capt, USAF, NC, MSN, APRN, NP-C, NRP
Nurse Practitioner, Family Medicine, Privileged Advanced Practice Nurse; Captain, United States Air Force, 5th Medical Operations Squadron, 5th Medical Group, 5th Bomb Wing, Minot Air Force Base, Minot AFB, North Dakota

LUCY MAYS, DNP, APRN, FNP-BC, CNE
Family Nurse Practitioner, St. Claire Regional Primary Care, Associate Professor of Nursing, Morehead State University, Morehead, Kentucky

MELANIE McGHEE, MSN, RN, ACNP-BC
St. Thomas Heart at St. Thomas West, Nashville, Tennessee

VANESSA MILLS, MSN, RN, CNL
Assistant Professor, The University of West Alabama, Livingston, Alabama

LYNN C. PARSONS, PhD, MSN, RN, NEA-BC
Professor and Department Chair, Department of Nursing, Center for Health, Education and Research, Morehead State University, Morehead, Kentucky

MARCIA A. PUGH, DNP, MBA, HCM, RN
Chief Nursing Officer, Bryan W. Whitfield Memorial Hospital, Tombigbee Healthcare Authority, Demopolis, Alabama

MARIA A. REVELL, PhD, MSN, RN, COI
Associate Professor and MSN Program Director, Division of Nursing, Tennessee State University, School of Nursing, Nashville, Tennessee

CHAD ROGERS, MSN, RN
Assistant Professor, Department of Nursing, Morehead State University, Morehead, Kentucky

MELISSA M. ROMERO, PhD, FNP-BC
Associate Professor, School of Nursing, Northern Michigan University, Marquette, Michigan

RICHARD ROVIN, MD
Marquette General Neurosurgery, UP Health System Marquette, Marquette, Michigan

DEBRA HENLINE SULLIVAN, PhD, MSN, RN, CNE, COI
Graduate Program, Core Faculty, College of Health Sciences, School of Nursing, Walden University, Minneapolis, Minnesota

MICHELE WALTERS, DNP, APRN, FNP-BC, CNE
Associate Professor of Nursing, Center for Health Education and Research, Morehead State University, Morehead, Kentucky

CHRISTOPHER A. WEATHERSPOON, APRN, MS, FNP-BC
Family Nurse Practitioner, Veteran Affairs, Tennessee Valley Health System, Fort Campbell, Kentucky; Contributing Faculty College of Health Sciences, School of Nursing Graduate Program, Walden University, Minneapolis, Minnesota

DEBORAH WEATHERSPOON, PhD, MSN, RN, CRNA
Core Faculty Leadership and Management Specialty, School of Nursing Graduate Program, College of Health Sciences, Walden University, Minneapolis, Minnesota

LIBRARY
FORSYTH TECHNICAL COMMUNITY COLLEGE
2100 SILAS CREEK PARKWAY
WINSTON SALEM, N.C. 27103

Contents

Health care is continuously undergoing evolutionary changes. These changes have been very dramatic for the end users. Instead of simple physician office visits and lengthy hospital stays, we are now faced with short hospital stays, office visits to different specialty providers, and an array of choices around them. With the present highway of choices between illness and wellness, it is important for transitions between these two to be affordable, advantageous to patients, and uncomplicated. This article discusses the choices patients and health care providers must make as the number of care options increase along with the risks and benefits.

Health care organizations must adopt a culture of safety and implement effective fall prevention protocols. The teach-back method is a useful strategy for health providers to determine patient understanding of information taught to maintain a safe environment and prevent falls. Purposeful rounding is a proactive approach to ensure that patient assessments are accurate and research supports that patients use the call light less when nurses participate in hourly rounding. This article provides the reader with evidence-based fall prevention interventions, tips for using the teach-back method, and fall prevention tools to safely care for patients of all ages.

Technology is rapidly changing the way nurses deliver patient care. The Health Information Technology for Economic and Clinical Health Act of 2009 encourages health care providers to implement electronic health records for meaningful use of patient information. This development has opened the door to many technologies that use this information to streamline patient care. This article explores current and new technologies that nurses will be working with either now or in the near future.

RECEIVED JAN 0 4 2016

At present there is a lack of well-validated surveys used to measure quality of life in patients with malignant brain tumors and their caregivers. The main objective of this pilot study was to validate the National Institutes of Health Patient-Reported Outcomes Measurement Information System (NIH PROMIS) survey for use as a quality-of-life measure in this population. This article presents the rationale for using the NIH PROMIS instrument as a quality-of-life measure for patients with malignant brain tumors and their caregivers.

Disruption in the interaction between the central nervous system, nerves, and muscles cause movement disorders. These disorders can negatively affect quality of life. Deep brain stimulation (DBS) has been identified as a therapy for Parkinson disease and essential tremor that has significant advantages compared with medicinal therapies. Surgical intervention for these disorders before DBS included ablative therapies such as thalamotomy and pallidotomy. These procedures were not reversible and did not allow for treatment adjustments. The advent of DBS progressed therapies for significant movement disorders into the realm of being reversible and adjustable based on patient symptoms.

Diabetes is a worldwide epidemic with a high cost regarding consumption of health care resources and is associated with high levels of morbidity and mortality. The complex nature of diabetes requires the use of evidence-based guidelines regarding diabetes management. These evidence-based guidelines are lengthy and do not readily translate into nursing care. As an integral component of the interprofessional team, the nurse must provide a thorough assessment of patients with diabetes and work to achieve individual patient treatment goals. Evaluation of patient progress toward treatment goals with regular/frequent follow-up is necessary to promote effective self-management of diabetes.

Aortic valve disease is a common and serious valvular disorder. Transcatheter aortic valve replacement is an option requiring nursing knowledge for the best patient outcome.

> Tobacco use contributes to the largest proportion of preventable disease, disability, and death. Use of tobacco products is at epidemic proportions in the United States. Estimates retrieved between 2012 and 2013 by the US Centers for Disease Control and Prevention reported that 1 in 5 adults used tobacco products. Tobacco use was greatest among men, young adults, those living in the Midwest and south, and those with less education. Cigarette smoking resulting in inhalation of tobacco and its by-products is the most common form of tobacco use. Tobacco use results in multiple diseases, including numerous cancers and chronic diseases.

> Bedside reporting continues to gain much attention and is being investigated to support the premise that "hand-off" communications enhance efficacy in delivery of patient care. Patient inclusion in shift reports enhances good patient outcomes, increased satisfaction with care delivery, enhanced accountability for nursing professionals, and improved communications between patients and their direct care providers. This article discusses the multiple benefits of dynamic dialogue between patients and the health care team, challenges often associated with bedside reporting, and protocols for managing bedside reporting with the major aim of improving patient care. Nursing research supporting the concept of bedside reporting is examined.

> Management of travel-related diseases acquired in Haiti begins with the identification of tropical diseases that are prevalent in the region. Knowledge of various tropical disease incubation periods and presenting symptoms is crucial to ensure rapid triage and management of care.

> This article presents a brief review and summarizes current therapies for the treatment of chronic obstructive pulmonary disease, major depression, and rheumatoid arthritis. One new pharmaceutical agent is highlighted for each of the topics.

> Peripheral intravenous (IV) access provides a means to administer medications, IV fluids, and blood products and allows for the sampling of blood for

NURSING CLINICS OF NORTH AMERICA

THE CLINICS ARE AVAILABLE ONLINE!
Access your subscription at:
www.theclinics.com

Foreword

Patient-Centered Care and Lifelong Learning

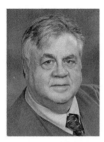

Stephen D. Krau, PhD, RN, CNE
Consulting Editor

The concept of "patient-centered care" has transitioned from a general notion to a focus that is in the forefront of health care delivery on many levels. Although there has been much discussion of what constitutes patient-centered care, benchmarks and evidence remain elusive. "Patient-centered care" is a phrase that has become an integral part of the lexicons of health care institutions, health care planners, congressional representatives, and hospital public relation departments.[1] The notion embodies the essential elements that patients are known in the context of their own communal worlds. Patients are informed, engaged in their care, and respected by the health care professional and the health care institution as their desires are seriously considered when involved with the health care environment. Even as the concept is prominent in the political agenda, measures and approaches to patient-centered care do not clearly demonstrate if, or to what extent, it is happening.[1]

With the many changes that have occurred in health care, the operational definition of patient-centered care is evolving and ever-changing. Measures to reflect these changes are influenced by many factors and have fallen behind. For example, early benchmarks for validating that the care patients received was patient-centered were based on the extent to which patients had the opportunities to ask questions.[1] This could be in the form of the patient being asked if he or she had any questions about the interaction or plan toward the end of the interaction. In an approach that is truly patient-centered, the patient should be invited to participate in the planning of care and the care should be tailored to the patient's level of needs. This mandates that health care professionals not only identify important aspects of the patient's societal world but also remain current in approaches and interventions to provide alternatives to care that are customized toward the patient's needs and desires.

Hudon and colleagues[2] discuss the measurement of patient-centered care and approaches that have been proposed to measure elements of patient-centered care to

Nurs Clin N Am 50 (2015) xi–xiii
http://dx.doi.org/10.1016/j.cnur.2015.10.002
0029-6465/15/$ – see front matter © 2015 Published by Elsevier Inc.

nursing.theclinics.com

| Table 1 |
| Interaction of elements related to patient-centered care |

Element	Relationship to Patient-Centered Care
Philosophy	Essentially, this approach to care is considered "the right thing to do." Within the confines of this view, patient-centered care is based on human respect and justice and is justified on the basis of moral grounds without regard to actual health outcomes.
Behaviors	Confusion related to this approach is the result of blending behaviors with outcomes. For example, the patient is satisfied with his or her health care interactions with the providers, but his or her health state actually declines. It becomes difficult to discern if the center of care is the result of the patient's perception of the interaction or the patient's actual health care outcomes. Models and studies between the relationship of patient-centered care and overall health care outcomes are just beginning to develop.
Outcomes	The conundrum of outcomes is the result of the common acceptance that the perception of the patient is the determinant as to what extent patient-centered care has occurred.
Health care professional knowledge	From the perspective of the health care professional, an essential element of patient-centered care is logically the knowledge and skills of the provider to assess, implement, and evaluate care. Without ongoing learning and professional development of the provider, the quality and purity of patient-centered care are stunted and compromised and present with limited options for a meaningful approach regardless of philosophy, behaviors, or outcomes.

Modified from Epstein RM, Street RL. The values and value of patient centered care. Ann Fam Med 2011;9(2):100–3; and Hudon C, Fortin M, Haggerty JL, et al. Measuring patient perceptions of patient-centered care: a systematic review of tools for family medicine. Ann Fam Med 2011;9(2):155–64.

develop research and produce evidence of its presence in various situations. The authors also point out the prominent ambiguity in measurement approaches that are greatly the result of confusion associated with philosophy, behaviors, and outcomes related to patient-centered care. Consideration of these elements is essential along with current knowledge to assure care that is patient-centered is occurring. **Table 1** presents a brief overview of these elements as they relate to patient-centered care.

As nurses take a lead in patient-centered care, they are required to be flexible and creative and critical thinkers to deliver safe and effective patient-centered care.[3] To this end, it is essential to engage and foster lifelong learning. This requires a commitment from nurses to accept and integrate education into their everyday practice.[3] Without preparation in current technologies, protocols, and treatment, patient-centered care cannot be complete, if it can occur at all. As identified by Parsons and Revell,[4] "it is important for the nurse to see care as a continuum and not finite." A requisite to patient-centered care is ongoing and a lifelong learning.

Stephen D. Krau, PhD, RN, CNE
Vanderbilt University Medical Center
309 Godchaux, 461 21st Avenue South
Nashville, TN 37240, USA

E-mail address:
steve.krau@vanderbilt.edu

REFERENCES

1. Epstein RM, Street RL. The values and value of patient-centered care. Ann Fam Med 2011;9(2):100–3.
2. Hudon C, Fortin M, Haggerty JL, et al. Measuring patient perceptions of patient-centered care: a systematic review of tools for family medicine. Ann Fam Med 2011;9(2):155–64.
3. Govranos M, Newton JM. Exploring ward nurses' perceptions of continuing education in clinical settings. Nurse Educ Today 2014;34(4):655–60.
4. Parsons L, Revell M. Preface: clinical updates in pathophysiology and care protocols for nursing management. Nurs Clin North Am 2015;50(4):xv–xvi.

Preface

Clinical Updates in Pathophysiology and Care Protocols for Nursing Management

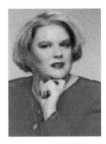   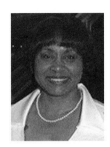

Lynn C. Parsons, PhD, MSN, RN, NEA-BC   Maria A. Revell, PhD, MSN, RN, COI
Editors

This issue of *Nursing Clinics of North America* shares new, cutting-edge information for delivering patient care for the person with varying disorders. Nursing is an evolving profession that requires continued knowledge updates in formulating a foundation for practice. In order to promote patient safety and satisfaction, it is imperative that nurses monitor publications and increase their knowledge base.

Specific patient care information and care protocols include cardiovascular disease, diabetes mellitus, orthopedic injuries, tobacco-related dependence, oncology management, peripheral vascular disease, congestive heart failure, movement disorders, and management of travel-related illnesses. Pharmacology updates, advances in treatment technologies, protocols for bedside reporting between nurses on a hospital unit, and care transitions across various health care organizations are addressed.

Each patient is different; each care management situation requires an individualized plan of care. These require the nurse to develop a personal framework for practice that continually develops from this information. This mandates an evolving knowledge base that this issue supplies for nurses who work to deliver care that is research-based and protocol-driven. This issue of *Nursing Clinics of North America* is both timely and relevant as it combines two clearly important topics for nurses in care management, pathophysiological updates as well as research-based protocols that are important to continuity of validated evidence-based care delivery. This will give nurses across organizations the opportunity to see care from a perspective of patient wholeness and not truncate care in order to address total components. With care reimbursement dependent on outcomes, it is important

Nurs Clin N Am 50 (2015) xv–xvi
http://dx.doi.org/10.1016/j.cnur.2015.10.001
0029-6465/15/$ – see front matter © 2015 Elsevier Inc. All rights reserved.

nursing.theclinics.com

for the nurse to see care as a continuum and not finite. This issue gives nurses this perspective.

Lynn C. Parsons, PhD, MSN, RN, NEA-BC
Center for Health, Education, and Research
Morehead State University
316 West Second Street
Suite 201P
Morehead, KY 40351, USA

Maria A. Revell, PhD, MSN, RN, COI
Tennessee State University
School of Nursing
3500 John Merritt Boulevard
Box 9590
Nashville, TN 37209, USA

E-mail addresses:
l.parsons@moreheadstate.edu (L.C. Parsons)
mrevell1@tnstate.edu (M.A. Revell)

Transitioning Care Across Various Health Care Organizations

Marcia A. Pugh, DNP, MBA, HCM, RN[a],*, Vanessa Mills, MSN, RN, CNL[b]

KEYWORDS

- Transitioning • Health care • Hospital • Choices • Electronic health record
- Care coordinator

KEY POINTS

- Changes in health care have brought many options for patients who are transitioning from one level of care to another that was previously unavailable.
- Each health care team member must take advantage of all opportunities for an improved outcome for patients.
- Transitioning care must be patient centered, starting with a patient-driven care plan.
- A care coordinator should be used to best overcome the many barriers to transitioning care. An electronic health care record should be used to facilitate transitioning care among all parties involved in the transition.

INTRODUCTION

As people live longer, they are apt to develop diseases that are more chronic and experience more complex disease processes, thus using more health care resources. The life expectancy in the United States was 78.7 years in 2011.[1] Although healthy aging is the goal, with an increase in years of life, the population is also at an increased risk of developing chronic age-related disorders. Managing these disorders requires planned health as well as social services. These services can include multimodal services in that hospital discharge often requires such follow-up care as outpatient rehabilitation and home health services. Pharmaceutical advances for disease treatment mean complex medication regimens, which can include multiple medications that must be administered several times a day.[2] These regimens can include medications that require training and skill to administer. There are options available that will help ease the transition from sickness to wellness, but there are also barriers to these

[a] Bryan W. Whitfield Memorial Hospital, Tombigbee Healthcare Authority, 105 Highway 80 East, Demopolis, AL 36732, USA; [b] The University of West Alabama, Brock Hall 206, 100 US-11, Livingston, AL 35470, USA
* Corresponding author.
E-mail address: mapugh1@gmail.com

Nurs Clin N Am 50 (2015) 631–643
http://dx.doi.org/10.1016/j.cnur.2015.07.003
0029-6465/15/$ – see front matter © 2015 Elsevier Inc. All rights reserved.

options. In order to maximize the benefit of available resources, the transition must be managed effectively and efficiently.

HEALTH CARE YESTERDAY

Initial health care saw the physician as the sole medical provider. In the late nineteenth and early twentieth centuries, the frontier doctor covered a large territory.[3] This general practitioner provided all of the medical treatments with no specialty education or equipment. There were no offices. With farms and settlements long distances from each other and no central doctor's office, the physician was most often expected to go to the person needing medical care. If care required intense treatment, this was done in the home with family and friends as caregivers. The physician visited the home as necessary to treat symptoms as they developed and assess treatment outcomes.

In the 1700s, central places for isolation of those with infectious diseases came into existence. These places were established in some US cities. Larger towns saw the founding of almshouses for the housing of not only the sick but also the poor, homeless, and destitute.[4] The mid 1700s saw the first institution established as a central place for provision of medical care for treatment of the sick.[5] This institution was known as a hospital where the sick and infirmed were cared for.

Since that time, hospitals have been used for treatment and convalescence. People were admitted to the hospital by the physician who determined the need for hospitalization, the specific treatment to be provided, as well as the length of stay. All necessary care was provided according to the physician's determined diagnosis and treatment no matter how lengthy or involved the procedure, diagnostic study, or the cost of such care. Even if the ordered medication could be administered in an outpatient setting, patients remained in the hospital with no questions asked.

There were few alternatives to hospitalization. The initial public health nurse made home visits to promote environmental health and safety. The end of the twentieth century saw the emergence of the public health nurse in the provision of individualized care.[6] However, the nurse was rarely used to give injections, change dressings, or perform patient assessments. Diagnostic studies that required a prep were done in the hospital, and there was no such thing as same-day surgery or outpatient surgery. There was no transitioning care. People had one physician, one hospital, and one pharmacy.

HEALTH CARE TODAY

As a society, we have moved to the opposite end of the spectrum. Today, there are many options available to the person who is not a candidate for hospitalization either because of the person's personal convictions or because the insurance policy warrants outpatient treatment. Today, hospitalization is for the acutely ill and only until the patients' condition improves, so further treatment can be safely provided in the home or outpatient setting.

There are many, many health care provider specialties and each one treats a particular part of the body. Acute health care can be obtained at a private physician's office, a specialty clinic, an emergency medical care facility, an urgent care/walk-in clinic, or community health center. In rural communities, the existence of these medical care requirements coupled with a lack of adequate transportation can present a hardship to patients. Overcoming such obstacles can require patients or caregivers to exert considerable effort in order to make appointments around their daily schedules and/or routines. Transitioning care in such instances can be vital in order to promote compliance.

Yesterday's inpatient surgical and specialty procedures are now performed as outpatient procedures. The options for outpatient services are varied in scope, practice, and complexity. Procedural preps previously performed in the hospital setting are now explained in detail by the health care provider and are expected to be carried out in the home setting. The associated procedures are performed in hospital outpatient care centers, specialty surgery centers (surgicenters), and specialty treatment centers (oncology, gastrointestinal, imaging, laboratory services, and rehabilitative services).

Postacute care can mean prolonged and extensive care. Preexisting conditions and age-related vulnerabilities, such as slowed healing processes, can make postacute care long, difficult, and laden with barriers and setbacks. A Centers for Medicare and Medicaid Services (CMS) 2011 study showed that 1 in 5 seniors on Medicare return to the hospital within a month of discharge.[7] A further study finalized in 2013 showed "Medicare spending is expected to increase by 79% between the years 2010 and 2020, caused, in-part, by hospital readmissions within 30 days of discharge."[8] For this reason alone, transitioning care is vital.

TRANSITIONAL CARE

"Transitional care refers to the patient moving from one care setting to another care setting and the actions required during that transition in order to provide continuity."[9] This transition must be designed to ensure continuity, fluidity, and coordination of care across all health care providers and services patients require. The transition must also be well communicated to each health care provider and to patients. A health care team that can consist of such health care providers as nurses, nurse practitioners, physician assistants, general practitioners, medical specialists, pharmacists, dietitians, palliative care specialists, rehabilitative personnel, and case managers. With the number of providers involved in patients' care, it is imperative that a plan be developed, that this plan is communicated among all health care providers, and that all involved, including the patients, understand the plan.

Transitions of care are not only interdisciplinary but are also intraorganizational (within organizations), interorganizational (among different organizations), and across health care types (curative to palliative and long-term care to home health). Assuring transitions among all care providers and organizations can prove to be an impossible task without the proper tools for development of a viable plan, responsible providers who are champions for success of the process, and informed and engaged patients.

THE PLAN

The transitional plan of care starts with the patients' diagnosis. With the aging population, multiple medical conditions often exist. Such multiplicity of chronic and acute health conditions requires continuous care management. For example, a person with a diagnosis of obesity can have other comorbid conditions, such as heart disease, type 2 diabetes, hypertension, gallbladder disease, osteoarthritis, sleep apnea and other breathing problems, and some cancers.[10] For this reason, when the health care provider indicates medical conditions exist, a plan of care should be initiated. This plan should be done regardless of the place where the primary diagnosis is made. The plan should be patient centered and should include the following:

- Medical diagnoses including all comorbidities
- Assessment of the patients' level of functioning (physical, psychosocial, cognitive, emotional)

- Financial (insurance) and economic status
- Support system
- Needed collaborative health care team members
- Education needed to inform patients, families, and/or caregivers of options to maintain up-to-date transitional care knowledge for informed decision making (**Table 1**)

THE HEALTH CARE PROVIDER

Each health care organization should have a staff person responsible for performing the task of transitioning care. Execution of the plan should be this person's ultimate responsibility. This person is the glue that ties the patients, health care providers, and health care organizations together into a plan that will ultimately provide the most effective resources that will help to ensure the best outcome for patients.

Communication is key. In order to ensure proper communication, the provider must be willing to spend the amount of time needed by patients to ensure dialogue on both sides.[11] **Table 2** identifies some problems that can exist in relation to communication and possible solutions.

The provider cannot be rushed or behave in such a way as to give the impression that the patients' opinion is not important. Rather than the provider allotting a specific amount of time to consult with patients, patients should be given the time needed to question the provider and to have their questions answered. The health care provider should ensure patients are given time to voice their concerns and there is acknowledgment and validation by the provider that patients have been heard.

There is to be a concerted effort made on the part of the provider to engage patients in conversation and to make patients feel they are in partnership with the provider in relation to the transition.[12] The conversation should be bilateral rather than unilateral. Patients should not feel they are being dictated to in relation to what is best and they should not be made to feel their choices are limited by the provider. Any suggestions or desires made known by patients are to be explored to the satisfaction of all parties.

Validation is an important part of communication. Validation means patients are understood and patients' views are accepted by the health care provider.[13] Acceptance of the patients' views does not mean there is agreement. Patients, as well as health care providers, have unique and individual views of how an effective transition should take place. Each party has their own views about what is appropriate care and even how much care is too much or not enough. There will sometimes be disagreements between the care patients want, feel is needed, and the care the health care provider feels is necessary for a transition. However, it is important that patients have a voice in the transition and that patients' wishes are granted if possible.

In order to validate patients' ideas and wishes, the health care provider should engage patients.[14] In order to engage patients in meaningful dialogue concerning the proposed transition, the health care provider must validate the situation, and the health care provider and patients must agree on what the situation is. Sometimes the two parties have very different views about the situation and how to resolve the situation to the satisfaction of all concerned parties. Engaging patients involves questioning, restatement of the situation, questioning again, and restating until both parties are satisfied. Only then can an effective and workable plan be devised.

PATIENTS

Patients must be the focus in all activities regarding transitioning care.[15] Patients must understand and be motivated to receive the health care options that are available. For

Table 1
Sample transitional plan of care

Interdisciplinary Activities	Assessment/Action
Diagnosis	Diabetes, morbid obesity, hypertension
Advance directives	Advance directive on file; do not resuscitate indicated
Health history	Type 2 diabetes, onset at 35 y of age Morbid obesity: reports gained 120 pounds over the last 5 y; eating reported as parental loss coping mechanism in 2010; hypertension diagnosis 3 y ago; bilateral total knee replacements (05/19/2015); no other surgeries
Allergies	None known
Level of functioning	Presently ambulating with great difficulty using walker States she is in pain level 10 when trying to ambulate Alert and oriented ×3
Insurance and benefits	Mills Commercial Insurance Company Copays: outpatient services, $250.00; office visits, $30.00; medications, $30.00; hospitalization, $1000.00; requires precertification for all outpatient and surgical procedures; home health, hospice, and durable medical equipment coverage
Living arrangements	Self-sufficient; capable of self-care and activities of daily living; lives alone; needs assistance during postrecovery period
Support system	Closest family members 50 miles away (name, relationship, address, and telephone number)
Communication	English primary language, conversational Spanish High school graduate Jehovah's Witness
Needed collaborative health care team members	Primary care physician, orthopedic surgeon, care coordinator, dietician, endocrinologist, pharmacist, physical therapist, home health care, pain clinic physician
Team member responsibilities	1. Patient: check blood sugar AC and HS, check blood pressure and weight weekly; record results in health journal 2. Home health nurse: to assess patient and perform dressing changes and assess healing process 3 times a week; specific wound care orders indicated 3. Home health aide: assistance with activities of daily living 4. Physical therapist: set up home exercise regimen and oversee exercises 3 times a week 5. Orthopedic surgeon: oversight of post–total knee care 6. Pain clinic: coordinate and oversee pain management regimen 7. Care coordinator: provide telephone support to promote cohesion between care providers 8. Patient: keep a journal and write down any questions about care to discuss with care coordinator
Diet	1800 cal ADA, low salt
Medications	Metformin 1000 mg po every 12 h Lisinopril 10 mg po daily Lortab 5 mg po every 4 h as needed for severe pain Acetaminophen 1000 mg po every 6 h as needed for pain

(continued on next page)

Table 1 (continued)	
Interdisciplinary Activities	**Assessment/Action**
Appointments	Dietician: (specify name, address, date, time and frequency) Endocrinologist: (specify name, address, date, time and frequency) Orthopedic surgeon: (specify name, address, date, time and frequency) Primary care provider: (specify name, address, date, time, and frequency) Pain clinic specialist: (specify name, address, date, time, and frequency)
Health education	Dietician to teach patient regarding diet; trainer to teach exercise regimen Pharmacist to teach correct administration and side effects of medication Physical therapist to teach home safety Home health nurse to teach home medication administration regimen and reinforce home safety Home health aide to teach bath safety and alternative methods for complete bath
Other	Care coordinator to provide telephone support 3 times a week

Abbreviations: AC, Latin "ante cibum", before meals; ADA, American Diabetes Association; HS, L. hora somni, before sleep, at bedtime.

example, if patients do not have a telephone in the home, then the use of telephonic care coordination would not be an option. The need for daily contact by a nurse to assess the patients' understanding of their medications, proper medication administration, and physical response to the medications being taken would need to be altered. If temporary cell phone acquisition is not a viable option, then talking to patients and caregivers would require their acceptance of home health care as an alternative.

Understanding the benefits of health care does not always ensure patients' desire or acceptance to receive the health care. Getting patients to recognize the need for a home health nurse does not guarantee acceptance or compliance. If home health care nursing is a part of the transitional plan because of the lack of telephone access capability and patients do not wish to have strangers in the home, then other options should be explored. One option would be to introduce the patients and caregivers to the home health nurse during an office visit. This meeting could allay the patients' fears of not knowing who is entering the home.

Table 2 Promotion of effective communication	
Problem	**Solution**
Ineffective communication	1. Ample time 2. Validate 3. Engage
Patients do not remember information	1. Patients repeat the information 2. Patients write the information
Patients cannot afford the recommended option	1. Use local services 2. Avoid redundancies

Problems arise when patients do not understand, do not remember, cannot afford services, or are not motivated or if orders do not agree with the plan for care transition. This circumstance often can be corrected with proper communication and assisting patients to become proficient in self-management.[16] There are transitioning care models available for specific patient populations; however, if patients are not the major influence in the transition, the transition will not provide the needed support. This means communication must occur between the providers and patients, but patients also have a responsibility to communicate preferences to the various providers.

BARRIERS TO TRANSITIONING CARE

Barriers to care relate to the health care provider, patients, and health care organizations. These barriers are not independent but interdependent. This topic is explained later.

Health care organizations tend to be independent providers. With the present payer systems, there is no incentive to transition care and promote care across different health care organizations or providers. Although some carriers promote managed care, there is no payment to encourage transitional care. As a patient is moved from provider to provider and health care organization to health care organization, each one is concerned with getting maximum payment for services provided in an effort to maintain their fiscal structure.[17]

The lack of interrelation communication, formal relationships, and collaboration can represent formidable barriers.[18] "A lack of communication between providers at hospitals, outpatient clinics, and home care agencies led to lack of continuity of care."[19] This development of a plan of care by one provider is not a consideration by another. Providers will often have their own independent plan of care that is specific to their particular treatment regimen. This plan can be influenced by marketing ancillary health providers. Often area specialty providers, such as hospices and durable medical equipment companies, court physician offices for referrals. Even pharmaceutical companies routinely visit physicians to leave samples and encourage use of their medications. These visits and freebies can influence the frequency of care as well as the quality of care. To ease financial burden, the physician might be likely to offer these samples in lieu of a prescription for a drug that is more beneficial to care of the patients.[20,21] Not only does this make patient education difficult, as patients may be taking a different drug to treat a specific condition with each office visit, it is not safe practice.

With care specificity and the number of available options for treatment and convalescence, problems can arise if the primary health care provider is not knowledgeable or does not understand the resources available to patients. The provider must thoroughly understand the resources patients need in order to communicate them to patients, to the patients' personal caregivers (family or paid caregivers), and to the patients' other health care providers. Using a care coordinator to manage patient transitions and assist patients with coordinating needed health care services can promote success.[22] The coordinator can keep updated resources and this information at hand. This coordinator can make care transition a smooth process.

Financial strain might mean patients may not be able to afford the health care associated with the transition. Health care providers do not always consider the expenses associated with possible health care transition options available to patients. Not only must health care providers consider the obvious cost of the treatment or service but also the time lost from work, traveling expenses, and sometimes the expense to family members or caregivers. Even with insurance, health care is a considerable expense.

As patients need providers, medications, therapies, and treatments that may accompany the transition, costs increase.

Defraying costs must be a part of the equation in relation to care transition if the transition is to be a success. There are ways the health care provider can assist patients. In order to defray costs, the provider would first look for local resources. There may be local clinics or treatment facilities that have specialists that come in periodically. Patients could see the specialist locally rather than traveling out of town. This option is especially beneficial in less populated towns that do not have access to certain services or specialists.

Another way to defray the high cost of health care associated with transitioning is to ensure services are not duplicated.[23] Duplicated services or care not only increase the cost to the patients but such duplications also waste resources and waste provider's time and the patients' time. In order to reduce cost, services could sometimes be combined. For example, if patients are to be transitioned from the hospital to home and are in need of home health care for wound care, assessments, patient and care giver education, physical therapy, and occupational therapy, then using one agency that can provide all needed services and coordinate home health care would benefit patients and promote care transition.[24]

To even further reduce the cost and promote care transition, the agency would have the same person provide the dressing change and the exercise rehabilitation. This practice would decrease the number of home visits, the amount of travel expense for the agency, and the number of personnel expended to the patients.

INFORMATION TECHNOLOGY AND THE ELECTRONIC HEALTH RECORD

In past years, the patients' medical health record was a hand written document kept in a file folder in a standard file cabinet. Patients completed demographic information and personal and family health history at each provider's office. Even if patients were referred to a specialty provider and parts of the medical record were shared, each office required completion of their particular forms. Although the initial assessment might have been accompanied by parts of that provider's medical record, once the care is provided, the specialty provider did not share their medical record. This situation meant that information could be conflicting or incorrect in that patients completed the documents from memory.

Each health care delivery provider generated his or her own record. One patient could have any number of records with several different health care providers and health service organizations in many different cities or even states. This situation can mean fractured care and conflicting care when the particular provider is given incorrect information provided by patients during provision of historical health information and previous health services,[25] which can be detrimental to any attempt to transition care when not all providers are known.

With the latest advances in computer technology, the patients' medical record is now electronic. The electronic medical record (EMR) is a digital version of the hard copy paper record previously kept in the physician's office. This record is maintained and managed by the physician's office to track and treat patients. It is specific to the patients' chief complaints and treatment history. This particular electronic program allows the provider to

- Track and monitor patient data over time
- Identify and schedule preventive screenings, immunizations, and check-ups
- Check and graph patient parameters, such as vital signs and blood glucose
- Monitor and promote health care performance improvement[26]

The electronic health record (EHR) is different from the EMR. This EHR can be used to overcome some of the barriers to transition. The EHR is designed to share information among different health care providers who are involved in the patients' care. This information is often created and managed by specified authorized providers and can be viewed and used by staff across different providers and organizations, which allows patient information to be shared and viewed among and across primary care providers, specialists, health care organizations, and others.

To promote the implementation and use of EMRs, both the CMS and individual state Medicaid programs have instituted EHR incentive programs.[27] With the federal government's regulations regarding the use of an EHR, there are very few providers not using at least some form or part of an EHR for their patients.[28] This point is true even if the physician office is using an EMR that is only accessible within their particular practice.

With real-time data entry, the patients' record is available and up to date at all times, which means that any provider of care could have immediate access to the most current information on patients. This practice promotes better-coordinated and efficient patient care.[29] The advantages of the implementation of the EHR are many. They include the following:

- Securely share health information with patients and other clinicians
- Effectively diagnose patients, reduce medical errors, and provide safer care
- Improve patient and provider interaction and communication as well as health care convenience
- Enable safer, more reliable prescribing
- Help promote legible, complete documentation and accurate, streamlined coding and billing
- Enhance privacy and security of patient data
- Help providers improve productivity and work-life balance
- Enable providers to improve efficiency and meet their business goals
- Reduce costs through decreased paperwork, improved safety, reduced duplication of testing, and improved health[30]

The patient information and technology are available to give patients access to their health care information. Patients can use this knowledge to facilitate transitioning and increase their control in the transition.[31] Patients should be given secure access to their diet plan, their medication regimen, and reminders for their appointments. As dietary recommendations change with a change in a laboratory value, patients can be given this information electronically in a securely accessed manner. If patients are not medically stable or competent to access their own record, then access should be provided to an in-home caregiver. When reports are added to the electronic chart, the health care provider has reviewed the report, and recommendations for a change in the plan of care are made, then an alert could be sent to the patients or caregiver. This trigger would provide an informational alert to look at the online information that has been added. With applications, this alert could be sent via a computer or smartphone. Secure access would afford review but not alteration of the patient record.

Health care providers sometime think patients should not know everything about their illness and/or prognosis. It has long been accepted by physicians that bad news would be depressing to patients and cause them to give up. Nurses strive to encourage patients without giving false hope. However, today, we know patients have a right to know everything about their diagnosis, treatment, and prognosis. If patients do not want to know everything, they should be able to choose how much of the record they can see, such as only their plan of care and instructions. Unless patients are very knowledgeable about managing their care, such as patients on dialysis who know what to do if their laboratory values change, then patients would only need access to their plan and instructions in order to transition effectively.

HEALTH CARE REFORM

There must be reform in health care in order to execute all activities necessary for effective transitional care. The reform must take place in the attitudes of health care providers.[32] Health care providers must resolve to allow more patient control and be open to actually striving to understand the patients' wishes. As nurses know, the best way to obtain patient compliance with any plan is to afford patients more participation in the planning of their care. For example, patients are much more likely to remember and abide by their dietary restrictions if they have met with the dietician and they, along with the dietician, have been able to determine a diet that patients can afford and incorporates some of the patients' desired dishes.

Health care providers must be mindful of the prevention of complications and begin expecting to provide prevention strategies as soon as a diagnosis is made. For example, patients who have been diagnosed with diabetes mellitus should immediately meet with a care coordinator who will assist with the necessary care transitions. Even though these patients might not be hospitalized, there will be a transition in care because they will need referrals to a dietician, an endocrinologist, and physical therapy for an exercise plan and other health care providers as certain risk factors might develop. Such initiation can be insurmountable in preventing possible complications.

Another way health care must reform is for insurance companies to agree to reimburse providers for proactive care.[33] Historically, insurance companies reimburse providers for care after a disease process has been determined and patients are ill. The insurance companies are reactive. In order to support transitional care, insurance companies will need to reimburse providers for such services as telephone communication, face-to-face communication with the care coordinator, and the full amount of time it takes for the communication. Insurance companies must also reimburse all wellness activities, such as wellness center visits, weight management endeavors, and other referrals made by the care coordinator.

INITIATING TRANSITIONAL CARE

Identifying the need for transitional care in the health care provider's environment means each person involved in the care of patients are cognizant of every opportunity to improve the patients' outcome by consulting the care coordinator. In an effort to promote prevention of complications and improvement in communication among the possible health care providers, the providers and organizations initiating transitional care should

1. Have a common mission in relation to transitional care. For example, maintain a communication health care network that would promote the highest level of wellness throughout the patient's care continuum.
2. Establish policies and procedures for health care providers performing transitional care and patients undergoing the transitions.
3. Provide education to the identified providers and organizations.
4. Establish quality- improvement initiatives for performance standards for care transitions.

5. Establish a system to monitor performance against these standards.
6. Identify a champion to promote the transition initiative.
7. Develop and build collaborative relationships among providers to promote ease of transitions among providers and organizations.[34]

SUMMARY

As defined by the American Geriatrics Society, transitional care is a set of actions designed to ensure the coordination and continuity of health care as patients transfer between different locations or different levels of care within the same location.[35] With shorter hospital stays and stricter insurance requirements for hospital admissions, hospitalization often means a higher acuity of illness. This circumstance coupled with the increased number of patients with chronic and acute complex medical conditions that can increase the number of health care professionals involved in the care can mean a perilous journey to wellness for patients. Transitioning care can promote compliance, allay fears in patient self-care management, empower patients and families, and promote quality health care. Proper care transitioning is rewarding to all involved and can ultimately improve outcomes, prevent readmissions to health care facilities, and decrease the cost of health care to patients and providers.

REFERENCES

1. Centers for Medicare and Medicaid Services. National vital statistics report. Atlanta (GA): National Vital Statistics System; 2012. p. 1–51.
2. Muir A, Sanders L, Wilkinson W, et al. Reducing medication regimen complexity. J Gen Intern Med 2001;16(2):77–82.
3. Oregon Health & Science University. Stories of frontier settlement doctors. 2012. Available at: http://www.ohsu.edu/xd/education/library/about/collections/historical-collections-archives/exhibits/frontier-settlement-doctors.cfm. Accessed May 15, 2015.
4. Nursing.upenn.edu. 1998. Available at: http://www.nursing.upenn.edu/nhhc/Welcome%20Page%20Content/History%20of%20Hospitals.pdf. Accessed May 17, 2015.
5. Graham KA. History of the Pennsylvania hospital. Charleston (SC): The History Press; 2008. p. 18–9.
6. Bekemeier B. Nurses on the frontlines of community health. Seattle (WA): Northwest Public Health; 2008. Available at: http://www.nwpublichealth.org/docs/nph/s2008/bekemeier_s2008.pdf. Accessed May 13, 2015.
7. Cms.gov. 2011-12-14-Centers for Medicare & Medicaid Services. 2015. Available at: http://www.cms.gov/Newsroom/MediaReleaseDatabase/Fact-Sheets/2011-Fact-Sheets-Items/2011-12-14.html. Accessed May 17, 2015.
8. DeCoster V, Ehlman K, Conners C. Factors contributing to readmission of seniors into acute care hospitals. Educ Gerontol 2013;39(12):878–87.
9. Coleman E. Commissioned paper: transitional care performance measurement. Performance measurement report. Institute of Medicine; 2006. p. 250–76. Appendix I.
10. Sampsel S, May J. Assessment and management of obesity and comorbid conditions. Dis Manag 2007;10(5):252–65.
11. Coulter A, Roberts S, Dixon A. Delivering better services for people with long term conditions: building the house of care. London: The King's Fund; 2013. p. 1–28.
12. Charles C, Whelan T, Gafni A. What do we mean by partnership in making decisions about treatment? BMJ 1999;319(7212):780–2.

13. Levinson W, Lesser C, Epstein R. Developing physician communication skills for patient-centered care. Health Aff 2010;29(7):1310–8.
14. Coulter A, Ellins J. Effectiveness of strategies for informing, educating, and involving patients. BMJ 2007;335(7609):24–7.
15. Naylor M, Stacen A. Transitional care: moving patients from one care setting to another. Am J Nurs 2008;108(9):58–63.
16. Warsi A, Wang P, LaValley M, et al. Self-management education programs in chronic disease. Arch Intern Med 2004;164(15):1641–9.
17. Woolhandler S, Himmelstein D. Correction: the deteriorating administrative efficiency of the U.S. health care system. N Engl J Med 1994;331(5):336.
18. Corrigan J. Crossing the quality chasm. Washington, DC: National Academies Press; 2005. Available at: http://www.ncbi.nlm.nih.gov/books/NBK22857/. Accessed May 22, 2015.
19. Dossa A, Bokhour B, Hoenig H. Care transitions from the hospital to home for patients with mobility impairments: patient and family caregiver experiences. Rehabil Nurs 2012;37(6):277–85.
20. Chimonas S, Kassirer J. No more free drug samples? PLoS Med 2009;6(5): e1000074.
21. Richardson D. Under the influence of drug companies. Br Columbia Med J 2009;51(1).
22. Bodenheimer T. Coordinating care — a perilous journey through the health care system. N Engl J Med 2008;358(10):1064–71.
23. Stewart B, Fernandes S, Rodriguez-Huertas E, et al. A preliminary look at duplicate testing associated with lack of electronic health record interoperability for transferred patients. J Am Med Inform Assoc 2010;17(3):341–4.
24. Coulter A, Roberts S, Dixon A. Delivering better services for people with long-term conditions: building the house of care. 1st edition. London: The KIngs Fund; 2013. Available at: http://www.kingsfund.org.uk/sites/files/kf/field/field_publication_file/delivering-better-services-for-people-with-long-term-conditions.pdf. Accessed May 21, 2015.
25. Jolt R, Los R, Bleeker S. Paper versus computer: feasibility of an electronic medical record in general pediatrics. Pediatrics 2006;117(6):15–21.
26. Garrett P, Seidman J. EMR vs EHR – What is the difference? - Health IT Buzz. Health IT Buzz. 2011. Available at: http://www.healthit.gov/buzz-blog/electronic-health-and-medical-records/emr-vs-ehr-difference. Accessed May 27, 2015.
27. Blumenthal D, Tavenner M. The "meaningful use" regulation for electronic health records. N Engl J Med 2010;363(6):501–4.
28. Hsiao C, Hing E, Socey T. Electronic health record systems and intent to apply for meaningful use incentives among office-based physician practices: United States, 2001–2011. 1st edition. Hyattsville (MD): National Center for Health Statistics; 2012. Available at: http://www.cdc.gov/nchs/data/databriefs/DB79.pdf. Accessed May 14, 2015.
29. Bates D. Getting in step: electronic health records and their role in care coordination. J Gen Intern Med 2010;25(3):174–6.
30. Healthit.gov. What are the advantages of electronic health records? | FAQs | Providers & Professionals | HealthIT.gov. 2015. Available at: http://www.healthit.gov/providers-professionals/faqs/what-are-advantages-electronic-health-records. Accessed May 27, 2015.
31. DeSalvo K. Building momentum: expanding patient access to medical records. Office of the Coordinator for Health Information Technology. 2013. Available at: http://www.healthit.gov/buzz-blog/consumer/building-momentum-expanding-patient-access-medical-records. Accessed May 24, 2015.

32. Fox A. Physicians as barriers to successful transitional care. Int J Adolesc Med Health 2002;14(1):3–7.

33. Naylor M, Sochalski J. Scaling up: bringing the transitional care model into the mainstream. 1st edition. New York: The Commonwealth Fund; 2010. Available at: http://www.wapatientsafety.org/downloads/TCM_Forefront.pdf. Accessed May 14, 2015.

34. Coleman E, Fox P. One patient, many places: managing health care transitions, part 1: introduction, accountability, information for patients in transition. Ann Long Term Care 2004;12(9):25–32.

35. Coleman E, Boult C. Improving the quality of transitional care for persons with complex care needs. J Am Geriatr Soc 2003;51(4):556–7.

Orthopedic Injuries

Protocols to Prevent and Manage Patient Falls

Lynn C. Parsons, PhD, MSN, RN, NEA-BC[a],[*],
Maria A. Revell, PhD, MSN, RN, COI[b],[1]

KEYWORDS

- Orthopaedic injuries • Fall prevention for children
- Fall prevention for adults and older adults • Joint Commission • Morse fall scale
- GRAF PIF risk assessment tool • Teach-back method • Protocols

KEY POINTS

- Participation in sports activities has increased for children and young adults over the past 20 years.
- The Joint Commission mandates assessment and reassessment for all hospitalized patients identified for fall risks.
- The General Risk Assessment for Pediatric Inpatient Falls is used for managing general risk and higher fall risks for pediatric patients.
- Hospitalized adults and older adult have several risk factors that can contribute to falls and sustaining injuries.
- The teach-back method is an effective model to determine the patients' level of understanding and to determine if learning took place.

Physical activity across the lifespan has a myriad of positive outcomes for children, adults, and older adults.[1] Participation in sports-related activities has increased for children and young adults in the past 20 years, yielding many benefits, including increased strength, dexterity, fitness, a sense of team play, and enhanced self-esteem. Structured weekly exercise classes for older adults support lower rates of falls, thereby reducing injury rates related to fracture.[2] The purpose of this article is to provide information for caregivers in structured hospital and health care settings

Disclosure Statement: The authors have nothing to disclose.
[a] Center for Health, Education and Research, Morehead State University, 316 West Second Street, Suite 201P, Morehead, KY 40351, USA; [b] Division of Nursing, Tennessee State University, 3500 John Merritt Boulevard, Box 9590, Nashville, TN 37209, USA
[1] 214 Jon Paul Court, Murfreesboro, TN 37128, USA.
* Corresponding author. 817 Greenfield Trail, Mount Sterling, KY 40353.
E-mail address: l.parsons@moreheadstate.edu

Nurs Clin N Am 50 (2015) 645–661
http://dx.doi.org/10.1016/j.cnur.2015.07.007   nursing.theclinics.com
0029-6465/15/$ – see front matter Published by Elsevier Inc.

that promote health, safety, and the prevention of injury and fractures related to patient falls.

PEDIATRIC CONSIDERATIONS

Children with skeletal abnormalities such as developmental dysplasia of the hip are at higher risk for injuries. In developmental dysplasia of the hip, gait is affected owing to different limb lengths that impact gait and agility in ambulation.[3] Other chronic pediatric disorders that adversely affect mobility include club foot, wherein 95% of diagnosed cases involve the foot being plantar flexed and inward, and osteogenesis imperfect, a rare condition of osteoporosis in children that involves bone fragility. Spinal deformity curves of 3 types—kyphosis, lordosis, and scoliosis—affects posture, balance, ambulation, and body image. Nurses caring for these children in hospital settings must provide a safe environment that minimizes the risk for falling and increased orthopedic injury.

Orthopedic injuries in sports-related activity are unavoidable with up to 40% of accidents taking place in recreational or competitive sporting events.[4,5] Prevention measures are challenging when you consider the large number of children participating in gym classes and school sports activities. Health professionals manage both acute and chronic musculoskeletal injuries in younger athletes.[6] Some young athletes participate in over 18 hours of athletic activities per week.[7] Monitoring of physical activities, caloric intake, and potential physiologic effects such as decreased sleep, fatigue, and overuse sports injuries must be assessed.[4,5] Children hospitalized owing to injuries or having injuries such as sprains and strains that require them to sit out on sports events interfere with the positive aspects of physical activity for active children and young athletes.

PEDIATRIC FALL PREVENTION

Children at risk for falling must be identified. Pediatric hospitals an inpatient pediatric units use various methods to determine fall risk.[8] A fall risk assessment must be done at admission and throughout the hospital stay. Nurses should asses the following risk factors for hospitalized children:

- Medication effects: postanesthesia or sedation; narcotic analgesics with special attention for children receiving these types of medications for the first time.
- Mobility issues: assess development age relative to ambulation, disease process, medical equipment such as casts, drains, or other adaptive equipment, especially if new for the patient.
- Fall history.
- Postoperative child: risk for postural hypotension, hypotension secondary to blood loss, medication effects and side effects, and specific health alterations such as musculoskeletal disorder.
- Infants or toddlers in crib or bed with side rails down.

PEDIATRIC FALL PRECAUTIONS

Fall risk tools are needed for the pediatric population to maintain a safe environment while hospitalized. Risks for falling are greater for ill hospitalized children versus well children in school or sports-related events. The Joint Commission mandates assessment and reassessment for patients identified at risk for falling.[9]

There are survey tools that provide risk assessment for falls in the pediatric population. The General Risk Assessment for Pediatric Inpatient Falls (GRAF PIF) tool was developed by Elaine Graf for use in the Children's Hospital in Chicago, Illinois.[9] The tool has since been adopted by many children's hospitals and inpatient pediatric units. The reader is referred to **Table 1** to view the 7 major assessment criteria and scoring process that highlights pediatric patients at greater risk for falling.

Each hospital organization can establish specific universal fall precautions unique to their pediatric population. The reader is referred to **Box 1** to view 1 organization's protocol for instituting pediatric fall precautions. Positive features of the GRAF PIF include:

- Fewer patients classified as high risk;
- Reduction of fatigue warnings;
- Increased opportunity for targeted interventions tailored to unit specific concerns; and
- Targeted educational programs for parents and family members.

A score of 2 or greater on the GRAF PIF identifies a pediatric patient at higher risk for a fall and nurses with a patient of a score of less than 2 would implement their organizations' standard precautions, which are also identified in **Box 1**. Infants younger than 12 months are automatically classified developmentally for a high risk of falling.[9] When the unit has greater numbers of high-risk patients for falling, additional staff support are required to assist with patient care. Hourly rounding and change-of-shift rounding and reports must include the fall status of the patient. The patient room should have clear walkways, the bed or crib in the lowest position with rails up, and the floor clear of cords, toys, linens, and any other items being used for the patient.

Table 1			
General risk for pediatric inpatient falls			
Risk Factor	**Item Score**		**Patient Score**
Length of hospital stay	1–4 d	0	—
	5–9 d	1	—
	≥10 d	2	—
IV/heparin lock	No	1	—
	Yes	0	—
PT/OT	No	0	—
(Recent past, current or expected in near future)	Yes	1	—
Antiseizure medication, given for any reason	No	0	—
	Yes	1	—
Acute or chronic orthopedic, musculoskeletal	No	0	—
Diagnoses	Yes	1	—
History of fall within past 1 month	No	0	—
	Yes	2	—
Fell during this hospitalization	No	0	—
	Yes	2	—
	Total score:		—

A score of 2 or greater is considered to be high risk.

Abbreviations: IV, intravenous; OT, occupational therapy; PT, physical therapy.

Data from Graf E. Identifying predictor variables associated with pediatric inpatient fall risk assessments. Proceedings from the 5th National Conference on Evidence-Based Fall Prevention. Clearwater, FL, March 29 – April 2, 2004.

Box 1
Protocol for universal fall precautions for all pediatric patients

- Institute universal fall precautions for all pediatric patients.
  - Universal precaution interventions related to patient education include:
    - Orient patient/family to surroundings;
    - Educate patient, family, and/or caregivers on falls safety while in the hospital;
    - Purpose and use of the call light;
    - Use of nonskid socks or well-fitting footwear;
    - Request assistance for daily activities (such as getting out of bed, toileting, transfers); and
    - Purpose and use of assistive devices and mobility aids, if needed.
  - Universal precaution interventions related to environment of care include:
    - Maintain call light within reach and is answered promptly;
    - Keep the patient's personal possessions within patient safe reach
    - Maintain bed in the lowest position when a patient is resting in bed unless staff is in attendance and providing care;
    - Place patient in appropriate crib/bed for developmental age;
    - Determine safest bedrail position and keep the upper rails and crib rails at maximum height when patient is in bed;
    - Keep hospital bed wheels locked;
    - Keep wheelchair wheels and recliners in locked position when stationary;
    - Keep patient care areas uncluttered;
    - Clean up spills immediately;
    - If patient wears glasses, ensure they are in place before ambulation; and
    - Follow safe patient handling practices and modify environment for safe transfers as needed.
  - Place yellow fall risk identifier on the patient's identification arm band.
  - Consider additional staff support when assisting patient.
  - Include falls status in daily rounding and nursing hand-off communication.

GRAF PIF Question 1: Length of Hospital Stay

1 to 4 days

5 to 9 days

10 or greater

GRAF PIF Question 2: IV/heparin lock

No

Yes

GRAF PIF Question 3: PT/OT recent past, current or expected in near future

No

Yes

GRAF PIF Question 4: Antiseizure medication, given for any reason

No

Yes

GRAF PIF Question 5: Acute or chronic orthopedic, musculoskeletal diagnosis

No

Yes

- Assist with transfer and mobility

GRAF PIF Question 6: History of fall within past 1 month

No

Yes

GRAF PIF Question 7: Fell during this hospitalization

No

Yes

- Place a yellow blanket with the patient and a yellow flag on patient's door frame. Educate patient and family/caregiver that the patient is at an increased risk for falls while admitted and the yellow helps everyone identify that fact and be more aware.

Other fall prevention interventions based on clinical judgment:

Abbreviations: GRAF PIF, General Risk Assessment for Pediatric Inpatient Falls; IV, intravenous; OT, occupational therapy; PT, physical therapy.

Courtesy of L. Wilson, DNP, MSN, RN, Chief Nurse Officer, St Claire Regional Medical Center, Morehead, KY; with permission.

The nursing staff will implement standard fall risk precautions for a score of less than 2. Standard fall precautions are implemented for children at low risk for falling while hospitalized. The following general interventions will be placed:

- Educate the parents, family members, and the patient on the importance of a safe, "fall-free" environment
- Orient the parents, family members, and patient to the room, where general supplies are located, bed devices, and call light system;
- Place the bed/crib in lowest position with the brakes on;
- Keep bed rails up;
- Keep crib rails up to the highest level;
- Wear nonskid slippers when walking; and
- Walk with a nurse, therapist, or family member as condition permits.

MAINTAINING SAFE ENVIRONMENTS IN HOSPITAL SETTINGS

Data support that a well-developed, research-based fall prevention program is needed; more than 28% of nonfatal injuries occur owing to falls.[10] The National Database for Nursing Quality Indicators defines a fall as an unplanned sudden descent, with or without personal injury, that results in the patient coming to rest on the floor.[11] In 2013, more than 30,000 deaths resulted in unintentional falls for persons of all ages, genders, and races in the United States.[12] Increased longevity and persons in the oldest-old age group, age 85 and older is the fastest growing segment of the US

LIBRARY
FORSYTH TECHNICAL COMMUNITY COLLEGE
2100 SILAS CREEK PARKWAY
WINSTON SALEM, N.C. 27103

population. Therefore, older adults are more likely to have chronic diseases such as osteoporosis and osteoarthritis that can increase the chance for falling, sustaining a fracture, and experiencing pain and loss of mobility. Health care costs for treating fall-related injuries are escalating and the Center for Medicare and Medicaid Services no longer reimburses hospitals for additional expenses related to injuries sustained after a fall. Health insurance companies could follow this practice in the future.

In health care settings, nurses must take the lead in identifying patients at risk for falling; however, interventions must be supported by all employees, including upper-level administrators. Health care agencies must develop a culture of safety and injury prevention. A comprehensive fall prevention plan must involve all employees, implementation of current evidence-based fall prevention interventions, and sound follow-up plans to continually improve quality care delivery (**Box 2**).

Purposeful hourly rounding is widely cited by many authors as a proactive approach in assessing the patient and the care setting.[13] Another positive finding in another investigation cited decreased call light use when nurses participated in hourly patient rounds.[14]

CARE OF THE ADULT AND OLDER ADULT

Prescribed medication contributes to the risk factors associated with adult and older adult patient falls as well. Certain categories of medications, such as psychotropics, antiemetics, barbiturates, and antidepressants, have side effects that alter sensorium and lead to confusion, drowsiness, loss of balance, and dizziness.[13,15] Patients receiving neurologic checks or being restrained need to be more closely monitored by nursing staff because they are at higher risk for falling. Nurse managers need to

---

Box 2
Major components for fall prevention programs

- Administrative support for a culture of safety.
- Medical staff leaders are integrated into the patient safety team.
- Strong interdisciplinary team members representing various professional groups; rehabilitation (physical therapy, occupational therapy), nursing, prescribing clinicians (physicians, midlevel providers), pharmacy, facilities and environmental services, managers and administrators, quality improvement, other key staff (volunteers, educators, dieticians, patient representatives, support staff such as secretaries and administrative assistants).
- Implementing fall prevention is a priority within the facility.
- Dedicated nonclinical time for interdisciplinary team meetings and activities.
- After a fall, review and root cause analysis.
- Updated policies and procedures for comprehensive fall prevention strategies.
- Continual review of current evidence-based fall prevention interventions.
- Implementation of current fall prevention protocols.
- Dedicated budget; assessment of current resources and identification of needed resources; examples could include adaptive equipment and environmental modifications.
- Assessment, development, and implementation for an orientation program for new and current employees (clinical and nonclinical).
- Visible role models and champions for fall prevention.

assess the registered nurse (RN) skill mix because these ratios are associated with increased likelihood of patient falls. Other nursing treatments needing to be closely monitored are pressure ulcer treatments; pain management and tube care were associated inversely fall risk. Use of laxative agents will lead to increased urgency for toileting. These patients need to be assisted to the toilet on a regular basis. Augmenting the RN staff mix with assistive personnel and placing patients closer to the nurses' station supports vigilant patient monitoring.

Essential to proficient fall risk assessment, patient safety and fall and injury/fracture prevention is a comprehensive evidence-based fall prevention and patient safety program that focuses on clinical and nonclinical staff. New employee orientation and ongoing staff development that includes discussion on safety and injury/fracture prevention must be acculturated within the workforce.[16] The reader is referred to **Box 3** to view how a hospital instituted universal precautions for all patients with special attention geared toward the adult and older adult.

EVIDENCE-BASED FALL PREVENTION PROTOCOLS

Hospitals and health care organizations such as long-term care facilities have formal protocols or policies or both to establish and maintain safety and prevent patient falls. Specific goals related to patient safety and defining important terms are helpful for employees to better understand role expectations.

The reader is referred to Appendix 1 to review an example of a hospital policy for evidenced-based fall prevention and patient safety program. Creating a culture of safety and providing patients within a therapeutic are the major goals of the policy and important terms are defined.

The Morse Fall Scale (MFS) is a simple method for assessing a patient's likelihood of falling; however, it is not a fall prevention tool.[17] A primary goal for the MFS is to identify why a patient is at risk for falling. Having this knowledge gives the interdisciplinary health team information needed to develop interventions to facilitate a safe environment that will decrease the probability for patient falls.[18] The MFS tool has 6 risk factor criteria:

- History of falling – if the patient fell within the past 3 months they have a score of 25.
- Secondary diagnosis – more than one medical diagnosis will score 15.
- Ambulatory aid – a patient using crutches/cane or walker will score 15; a patient walks clutching to furniture, does not ask for help when needed or is noncompliant with bed rest will score 30.
- Intravenous (IV)/saline lock - patient will score 20 if either device used.
- Gait – weak (stooped but can lift head and maintain balance; short steps, shuffling gait, uses furniture as a guide scores a 10); a patient with greater impaired gait will score a 20.
- Mental status – a patient who overestimates abilities or is forgetful will score a 15.

The reader is referred to **Table 2** to view the MFS that was adapted by a hospital for use with their adult patient population.

TEACH-BACK METHOD

The teach-back is a model that health educators use to assess for lapses in recall and understanding to reinforce patient teaching that has been done and support continuous engagement in communicating the importance of safety and fall prevention to hospitalized patients and their family. RNs should use the teach-back method to

Box 3
Universal fall precautions for all patients

- Institute universal fall precautions for all patients.
  - Universal precaution interventions related to patient education include:
    - Orient patient/family to surroundings;
    - Educate patient, family, and/or caregivers on falls safety while in the hospital;
    - Purpose and use of the call light;
    - Use of nonskid socks or well-fitting footwear;
    - Request assistance for daily activities (such as getting out of bed, toileting, transfers); and
    - Purpose and use of assistive devices and mobility aids, if needed.
  - Universal precaution interventions related to environment of care include:
    - Maintain call light within reach and is answered promptly;
    - Keep the patient's personal possessions within patient safe reach;
    - Maintain bed in the lowest position when a patient is resting in bed unless staff is in attendance and providing care;
    - Determine safest bedrail position, keep upper rails and crib rails at maximum height when patient is in bed;
    - Keep hospital bed wheels locked;
    - Keep wheelchair wheels and recliners in locked position when stationary;
    - Keep patient care areas uncluttered;
    - Clean up spills immediately;
    - If patient wears glasses, ensure they are in place before ambulation; and
    - Follow safe patient handling practices and modify environment for safe transfers as needed.
- Include falls status in daily rounding and nursing hand-off communication.

Morse Question 1: Do you have a history of falling in the past 3 months?

No

Yes

- History of injury with prior falls?
  No
  Yes- Injury without fracture
  Yes- Injury with fracture

- Location of fracture:
  Hip
  Wrist
  Shoulder
  Other: _____

- Other pertinent fall history:

- Reinforce need for assist/supervised transfers and mobility

Morse Question 2: Is the patient on multiple medications to manage multiple comorbidities?

No

Yes

- On medications that increase a patient's risk for falling or a risk for injury with falls?
  - Diuretics
  - Sedatives

- ○ Opioids
- ○ Hypnotics
- ○ Analgesics
- ○ Psychotropic
- ○ Antihypertensives
- ○ Antidepressants
- ○ Anticoagulants (increased bleed risk)
- ○ Other: _____
- Reinforce physician instructions for prevention of complications related to medical diagnosis.
- Review medications with patient and family/caregiver and take into account risks specific to the patient.
- Evaluate for orthostasis.
- Complete surveillance rounds every:
  - ○ 15 minutes.
  - ○ 30 minutes.
  - ○ 1 hour.
  - ○ 2 hours.
- Encourage/assist toileting before fall risk medication administration.

Morse Question 3: At baseline, patient uses ambulatory aids for mobility?

Straight cane

Quad cane

Rolling walker

Standard walker

Other: _____

- Assess that patient uses the device safely.
- Determine if patient is safe to have access to device at all times.

Morse Question 4: Does the patient have an IV, heparin lock, or saline lock?

No

Yes

- Provide patient and family/caregiver education regarding tubing as a tripping hazard and the effects of specific patient IV medications.
- Keep IV pole on the side the patient will exit the bed.

Morse Question 5: Does the patient have gait and/or transferring problems?

No: Normal

No: Bedrest or immobile

Yes: weakness

Yes: impaired

- Assist with mobility:
  - ○ Remind patient to call for assistance before attempting mobility.
  - ○ Use a gait belt and safe patient handling techniques to assist patient.
  - ○ Create a "safe exit side" for transfers from the bed.
  - ○ Ensure nonskid socks are used in mobility.
- Assist in toileting:
  - ○ Remain with patient during toileting.
  - ○ Provide bedside toileting devices if needed (ie, urinal, bedside commode).

- If patient has a new gait/transfer problem that effects functional mobility, consider consult to physical therapy for further evaluation.

Morse Question 6: Mental status

Oriented to own ability/knows own limitations.

Overestimates/forgets limitations.

- Reeducate/reminders regarding safety.
- Move closer to nurses' station.
- Bed/chair alarms as a reminder to call for assistance.
- Arrange for diversional activities.
- Encourage family/caregiver to visit with patient.

Other fall prevention interventions based on clinical judgment:

- Take orthostatic vitals.
- If patient is admitted owing to a fall or they have fallen during this admission, place a yellow blanket with the patient, a yellow flag on patient's door frame, and yellow arm bracelet snap. Educate patient and family/caregiver that the patient is at an increased risk for falls while admitted and the yellow helps everyone identify that fact and be more aware.

Abbreviation: IV, intravenous.

Courtesy of L. Wilson, DNP, MSN, RN, Chief Nurse Officer, St Claire Regional Medical Center, Morehead, KY; with permission.

ensure that learning and understanding have occurred. This system assesses the patient and/or their family members' ability to recall and reiterate what has been learned in their own words.[19] To confirm patient and family members' understanding of a fall prevention program, nurses should ask questions like, "What type of slippers are safe to wear?" and "What is the first thing to do before you attempt to get out of bed?" Many times, a person will respond that they understand to please the provider when asked a close-ended question such as, "Do you understand the information that I just shared?" The teach-back method has been endorsed by the National Quality Forum as a confirmed strategy in determining patient understanding when teaching hospitalized adults.[20]

The teach-back method has been found effective for low-literacy patients' with chronic medical conditions and their adherence to treatment.[20] The reader is referred to **Box 4** to view how a hospital uses the teach-back method to determining patient and family understanding of their fall prevention program.

When using teach back, the nurse should explain needed information to the patient or family caregiver and then ask in a nonshaming way for the individual to explain what he or she understood. For example, "I want to be sure that I did a good job of teaching you about staying safe from falling in the hospital. Can you please tell me in your own words how you can prevent falling?" If the staff member identifies a gap in understanding, he or she should offer additional teaching or explanation, followed by a second request for teach back to assess patient understanding for safety associated with the fall prevention program.

Table 2
Morse Fall Scale for identifying fall risk

Risk Factor	Item Score		Patient Score
1. History of falling (immediate or previous 3 months)	No	0	—
	Yes	25	
2. Secondary diagnosis (≥ 2 medical diagnosis in chart)	No	0	—
	Yes	15	
3. Ambulatory aid	None/bedrest/wheelchair/nurse	0	—
	Crutches/cane/walker	15	
	Furniture	30	
4. IV/saline lock	No	0	—
	Yes	20	
5. Gait/transferring	Normal/bedrest/immobile	0	—
	Weak[a]	10	
	Impaired[b]	20	
6. Mental status	Oriented to own ability	0	—
	Overestimates or forgets limitations	15	
	Total score[c]:		

Scores of <25 indicated low risk; 25–45, moderate risk; and >45, high risk.

[a] Weak gait: Short steps (may shuffle), stooped but able to lift head while walking, may seek support from furniture while walking, but with light touch (for reassurance).

[b] Impaired gait: Short steps with shuffle; may have difficulty arising from chair; head down; significantly impaired balance, requiring furniture, support person, or walking aid to walk.

[c] Suggested scoring based on Morse JM, Black C, Oberle K, et al. A prospective study to identify the fall-prone patient. Soc Sci Med 1989;28(1):81–6. However, note that Morse herself said that the appropriate cut-points to distinguish risk should be determined by each institution based on the risk profile of its patients. For details, see Morse JM, Morse RM, Tylko SJ. Development of a scale to identify the fall-prone patient. Can J Aging 1989;8:366–7.

From Agency for Healthcare Research and Quality (AHRQ). Preventing falls in hospitals – a toolkit for improving quality of care. Rockville (MD): 2013. Available at: http://www.ahrq.gov/professionals/systems/hospital/fallpxtoolkit.pdf. Accessed June 3, 2015.

Return demonstration is another method for closing the information loop. When using this technique, the nurse asks the patient to demonstrate how he or she will perform the action that was just explained. Many teams successfully used the technique to improve patient understanding and use of the call light.

Box 4
Tips for using teach back to redesign patient teaching

Use teach back with patients to improve understanding of:

- The reasons that the patient is at risk for falling and/or injury;
- The reasons fall prevention is important;
- Actions the patient can take to stay safe;
- The importance of patients asking for help when accessing the bathroom;
- The location and use of the call light; and
- The importance of using nonslip footwear.

SUMMARY

Health providers must have vigilant policies and health care protocols in place to promote patient safety, prevent patient falls, and decrease injuries for patient across the lifespan that are admitted to long-term care facilities and hospitals. Health care executives, medical staff, health care professionals, and nonclinical employees must embrace a culture of safety and be actively involved in interventions that decrease fall risk and injuries to patients.

Tools for pediatric and adult patients ameliorate safety interventions in health care organizations. Policies and protocols must be developed and continually reviewed and edited by each institution to best addresses the unique patient needs. The Joint Commission mandates that organizations have in place assessment tools for determining and managing patient fall assessment risk. Focusing on patient safety enhances quality care delivery and patient outcomes while addressing escalating health costs associated with patient falls.

REFERENCES

1. Maffulli N, Longo UG, Spiezia F, et al. Sports injuries in young athletes: long-term outcome and prevention strategies. Phys Sports Med 2010;2(38):29–34.
2. Wurzer B, Waters DL, Hale LA, et al. Long-term participation in peer-led fall prevention classes predicts lower fall incidence. Arch Phys Med Rehabil 2014;95: 1060–6.
3. Ortiz-Neira CL, Paulucci EO, Donnon T. A meta-analysis of common risk factors associated with the diagnosis of developmental dysplasia of the hip in newborns. Eur J Radiol 2012;81(3):e344–51.
4. Caine DJ, Maffulli N. Epidemiology of children's individual sports injuries. An important area of medicine and sports science research. Med Sport Sci 2005; 48:1–7.
5. Caine DJ, Nassar L. Gymnastics injuries. Med Sport Sci 2005;48:18–58.
6. Shanmugam C, Maffuli N. Sports injuries in children. Br Med Bull 2008;86:33–57.
7. D'Hemecourt P. Overuse injuries in the young athlete. Acta Paediatr 2009;98: 1727–8.
8. Child Health Corporation of America. Pediatric falls: state of the science. Pediatr Nurs 2009;35(4):227–31.
9. Graf E. Identifying predictor variables associated with pediatric inpatient fall risk assessments. Proceedings from the 5th National Conference on Evidence-Based Fall Prevention. Clearwater, FL, March 29 – April 2, 2004.
10. Shuey KM, Balch C. Fall prevention in high-risk patients. Crit Care Nurs Clin North Am 2014;26(4):569–80.
11. Montalvo I. The National Database of Nursing Quality Indicators (NDNQI). OJIN The Online Jrnl of Iss in Nsg 2007;12(3). Manuscript 2.
12. WISQUARS. Fatal injury reports, national and regional, 1999-2010. Available at: http://webappa.cdc.gov/sasweb/ncipc/mortrate10_us.html. Accessed June 3, 2015.
13. Boushon B, Nielsen G, Quigley P, et al. How-to guide: reducing patient injuries from falls. Cambridge (MA): Institute for Healthcare Improvement; 2012. Available at: www.ihi.org. Accessed June 2, 2015.
14. Olrich T, Kallman M, Nigolian C. Hourly rounding: a replication study. Medsurg Nurs 2012;21(1):23–6, 36.
15. Titler M, Shever L, Kanak M, et al. Factors associated with falls during hospitalization in an older adult population. Res Theory Nurs Pract 2011;25(5):127–48.

16. Agency for Healthcare Research and Quality (AHRQ). Preventing falls in hospitals – a toolkit for improving quality of care. 2013. Available at: http://www.ahrq.gov/professionals/systems/hospital/fallpxtoolkit/fallpxtoolkit.pdf. Accessed June 3, 2015.
17. Morse JM. Enhancing the safety of hospitalization by reducing patient falls. Am J Infect Control 2002;30:376–80.
18. Morse J. Preventing patient falls. Washington, DC: Sage; 1997.
19. White M, Garbez R, Carroll M, et al. Is "teach-back" associated with knowledge retention and hospital readmission in hospitalized heart failure patients? J Cardiovasc Nurs 2013;28(2):137–46.
20. National Quality Forum. Safe practices for a better healthcare – 2010 update. A consensus report. Available at: http://www.qualityforum.org/News_And_Resources/Press_Kits/Safe_Practices_for_Better_Healthcare.aspx. Accessed June 3, 2015.
21. Ganz DA, Huang C, Saliba D, et al. Preventing falls in hospitals: a toolkit for improving quality of care (Prepared by RAND Corporation, Boston University School of Public Health, and ECRI Institute under Contract No. HHSA2902010000171 TO #1). Rockville (MD): Agency for Healthcare Research and Quality; 2013. AHRQ Publication No. 13-0015-EF.
22. Rutherford P, Nielsen GA, Taylor J, et al. How-to guide: improving transitions from the hospital to community settings to reduce avoidable rehospitalizations. Cambridge (MA): Institute for Healthcare Improvement; 2012. Available at: http://www.ihi.org/knowledge/Pages/Tools/HowtoGuideImprovingTransitionstoReduceAvoidableRehospitalizations.aspx.
23. Meade CM, Bursell AL, Ketelsen L. Effects of nursing rounds: On patients' call light use, satisfaction, and safety. Am J Nurs 2006;106(9):58–70.
24. Oliver D, Healey F, Haines TP. Preventing falls and fall-related injuries in hospitals. Clin Geriatr Med 2010;26(4):645–92.

APPENDIX 1: EVIDENCE-BASED FALL PREVENTION AND PATIENT SAFETY POLICY

Policy

St. Claire Regional Medical Center is committed to establishing and maintaining an ongoing safety and fall prevention program that integrates evidence based guidance for clinical interventions and education to enhance caregivers' compliance and accountability.

Goals

Foster a culture of safety where care is provided. Place patients in the very best therapeutic and safe environment.

Purpose

To promote patient safety by:
A. Initiating universal fall precautions on all patients as a standard of care.
B. Routinely completing a validated fall risk assessment and identifying intrinsic or extrinsic factors that may place the patient at risk for falls.
C. Developing an individualized care plan as related to falls including preventive and protective interventions.

Definitions:

A *patient fall* is a sudden, unintentional descent, with or without injury to the patient, that results in the patient coming to rest on the floor, on or against some other surface (eg, a counter), on another person, or on an object (eg, a trash can; National Database for Nursing Quality Indicators, June, 2014).

Assisted fall: A fall in which *any staff member (whether a nursing service employee or not)* was with the patient *and* attempted to minimize the impact of the fall by slowing the patient's descent. Assisting the patient back into a bed or chair *after* a fall does not make the fall an assisted fall.

Unassisted fall: A fall in which *any staff member (whether a nursing service employee or not)* may or may not be present, but the patient's descent was *not* slowed. This is could also be an assumed fall, such as a patient found in the floor, in which no one witnessed the fall. A fall in which the family or visitor reported to assist the patient also represents an unassisted fall.

All assisted and unassisted falls can be further classified as:

A. Accidental falls: A fall owing to environmental factors in which the patient is cared for, especially because this is usually an unfamiliar environment to the patient. For example, suboptimal chair height, unsafe staffing levels, floor spills, furniture clutter, and poor lighting can all contribute to an accidental fall.

B. Anticipated physiologic falls: A fall that occurs in patients who have risk factors for falls that can be identified in advance, such as altered mental status, abnormal gait, frequent toileting needs, visual impairment, dementia, delirium, or high-risk medication. A standardized screening tool aims to identify these risk factors.

C. Unanticipated physiologic falls: A fall that occurs because of a sudden physiologic event whose timing could not be anticipated, such as seizure, syncopal episode, unexpected orthostatis, extreme hypoglycemia, stroke, or heart attack.

D. Baby/child drop: A fall in which a newborn, infant, or child being held or carried by a health care professional, parent, family member, or visitor falls or slips from that person's hand, arm, lap, or other grasp. This can occur when a child is being transferred from 1 person to another. This is counted as a fall regardless of whether an injury occurred.

E. Falls during play: Some units have psychiatric and pediatric gyms or play areas. Falls that occur during normal play activities in such areas should be reported only when an injury occurs.

I. St. Claire Regional Medical Center uses published evidence to offer a best practice approach for preventing falls in hospitals, including 4 key components.
   A. Implementation of a safe environment of care for all patients.

   a. Universal fall precautions.
   B. Identification of specific modifiable fall risk factors.

   a. Standardized fall screening tool for patients 12 months and older.

   i. Morse in the adult population.

   ii. GRAF PIF in the pediatric population.

   b. All infants less than 12 months are considered developmentally a high risk for falls.
   C. Implementation of interventions targeting those risk factors so as to prevent falls.
   D. Interventions to reduce the risk of injury to those people who do fall.

II. Fall prevention interventions are to be initiated and maintained for all patients.[21]
   A. Universal fall precautions.

   a. Apply to all patients at all times, regardless of their fall risk.

   b. Universal precautions revolve around patient education and keeping the patient's environment safe and comfortable.

   c. Universal precaution interventions related to patient education include:

   i. Orient patient/family to surroundings;

   ii. Educate patient, family, and/or caregivers on falls safety while in the hospital;

      iii. Purpose and use of the call light;

      iv. Use of nonskid socks or well-fitting footwear;

      v. Request assistance for daily activities (such as getting out of bed, toileting, transfers); and

      vi. Purpose and use of assistive devices and mobility aids, if needed.

  d. Universal precaution interventions related to environment of care include:

      i. Maintaining call light within reach and is answered promptly;

      ii. Keeping the patient's personal possessions within patient safe reach;

      iii. Maintaining bed in the lowest position when a patient is resting in bed unless staff is in attendance and providing care;

      iv. Determining the safest bedrail position—keep upper rails and crib rails at maximum height when patient is in bed;

      v. Keeping hospital bed wheels locked;

      vi. Keeping wheelchair wheels and recliners in locked position when stationary;

      vii. Keeping patient care areas uncluttered;

      viii. Cleaning up spills immediately;

      ix. If patient wears glasses, ensuring they are in place before ambulation; and

      x. Following safe patient handling practices and modify environment for safe transfers as needed.

  e. Use educational materials to teach fall prevention techniques, any fall interventions currently in place regarding the patient's fall risk factors, and what they can do to help prevent a fall. Encourage teach-back education in which the patient or family recalls and restates, in their own words, the information they heard during education.[22]

B. Purposeful hourly rounding on all patients.

  a. Hourly rounds are an opportunity to ensure that universal fall precautions are implemented and that patients' needs are being met.[23]

  b. These rounds integrate fall prevention activities with the rest of a patient's care.

  c. It should include the "5 P's":

      i. Pain: Assess the patient's pain level. Provide pain medicine if needed.

      ii. PO: Offer hydration, offer nutrition

      iii. Position: Help the patient get into a comfortable position or turn immobile patients to maintain skin integrity

      iv. Potty: Offer to assist to the restroom, bedside commode, or use the urinal. Empty commodes and urinals.

      v. Prevent falls: Ask patient/family to use call light if patient needs to get out of bed; consider universal fall precautions. Make sure patient's essential needs (call light, phone, reading materials, glasses, tissues, etc) are within easy reach.

  d. Documentation of interventions should be noted in the patient's record.

C. Complete the standardized fall screening tool on all hospital setting patients older than 12 months at admission, upon transfer from 1 unit to another, after a significant change in patient's condition, and after a fall or a near fall has occurred.

  a. Adults. The Morse Falls Scale (MFS) has established reliability and validity in the adult population. It is made up of 6 subscales:

      i. History of falls

      ii. Secondary diagnosis

      iii. Ambulatory aid

      iv. IV/heparin lock

      v. Gait

      vi. Mental status

   b. The total MFS score provides an indication of the likelihood that a patient will fall. A patient's fall risk can range from 0 to 125.

      i. Less than 25: Low risk

      ii. 25–45 Moderate risk

      iii. Greater than 45: High risk

   c. Pediatric. The General Risk Assessment for Pediatric Inpatient Falls (GRAF PIF) is currently validated for use with pediatric inpatients, ages 12 months through 16 years old. The GRAF PIF has 7 subscales:

      i. Length of hospital stay

      ii. IV/heparin lock

      iii. PT/OT

      iv. Antiseizure medication, given for any reason

      v. Acute or chronic orthopedic/musculoskeletal diagnosis

      vi. History of fall within past 1 month

      vii. Fall during this hospitalization

   d. A pediatric patient's fall risk can range from 0 to 10. A total score of 2 or greater indicates a high fall risk.

   e. Infants. All patients less than 12 months old are considered developmental high risk for falls.

   f. Situational events may place a patient at a high risk for a short period of time: Preoperative medications, preparation for diagnostic testing, postoperative procedures, cardiac catheterizations, etc.

D. The screening tool helps to identify risk factors for falling. Once specific risk factors are identified for a patient, further in-depth assessment needs to be completed to identify common reversible risk factors. These include delirium, postural instability, visual impairment, culprit medication, postural hypotension, syncope, urinary incontinence and frequency, behavioral disturbance, and agitation.[24]

   a. Nursing initiates focused interventions to improve a patient's reversible risk factors and creates a multifaceted fall care plan for the patient.

E. Outpatient and ancillary service areas will use the patient's past medical history, present medical condition, and visual cues to identity at risk patients and use safety measures for prevention. Transporters or designated person in the ancillary/diagnostic imaging department may be asked to stay with the patients until the testing is complete.

III. If the patient has a fall or near fall, with or without injury:

A. The staff member discovering the fall will attend to the patient's immediate needs. Staff provide immediate care and assist the patient to a level of comfort.

B. A nurse will assess the patient immediately.

C. The immediate care provider, nurse manager, and charge nurse along with the patient in the area of the fall will perform a post fall debriefing immediately after the fall. Complete the postfall analysis/assessment form and forward to nursing administration for distribution. The goal is to identify a root cause to the fall.

   a. Assess intrinsic and extrinsic factors that may have contributed to the fall. Note the circumstances: location, activity, time of day, and any significant factors/symptoms the patient experienced.

   b. Review any contribution factors, such as underlying illness, medications, functional or sensory deficits and psychological status.
D. The nurse will complete the standardized screening tool, reassess the patient's fall risk and initiate newly identified fall preventive measures.
E. After the fall, the patient, caregiver and family will receive additional training on fall risk status in the hospital. For the patient who is a known fall risk, this admission is identified with a yellow blanket, yellow flag at the door frame, and yellow fall risk identifier placed on the patient's arm band.
F. Pharmacy consultation for medication-related risk factors will be ordered in Meditech after a fall has occurred.
G. Physical therapy for fall risk factors will be ordered in Meditech after a fall has occurred.
H. The attending physician will be promptly notified by an RN to determine the need for further evaluation or orders.

   a. Communicate the modified plan of care to all caregivers.
I. An RN notifies the patient's family that a fall has occurred.
J. Documentation

   a. Document the episode of the fall, note any injury, physical assessment data, and implementation of post fall interventions in the patient medical record.

   b. Identify the event as a fall only if witnessed. If unwitnessed, state that the patient was found on the floor and what the patient tells you happened. Do not assume, speculate, or express an opinion.

   c. Complete a fall incident report in Meditech. Do not reference in the patient's medical record that an incident report was completed.
K. If the fall results in an unexpected occurrence involving death or serious physical injury, notify the chief nursing officer and risk management immediately.

IV. Staff who may assist with the ambulation or movement of patients will receive training on safe patient handling, falls, and fall prevention during orientation and on an annual basis. This skill will be considered as a component of the annual competency program.

V. Patient falls will be reviewed routinely by the falls subcommittee. The nurse manager and staff with the most knowledge concerning each fall will evaluate and present to the falls subcommittee routinely with an action plan for fall prevention. The falls subcommittee will report to the nurse quality council. Any identified trends or issues will be forwarded to the nursing executive council for review.

VI. The fall prevention program will be monitored, evaluated and reviewed on an annual basis by the falls subcommittee and the nurse quality council.

Courtesy of L. Wilson, DNP, MSN, RN, Chief Nurse Officer, St Claire Regional Medical Center, Morehead, KY; with permission.

Technological Advances in Nursing Care Delivery

Debra Henline Sullivan, PhD, MSN, RN, CNE, COI

KEYWORDS

- Electronic health records • Technology in nursing • Telehealth • Mobile technology

KEY POINTS

- Meaningful use incentives are encouraging health care organizations to implement electronic health records.
- Electronic health records are leveraging and encompassing new technologies.
- Nurses will be working in a high tech environment and must use these resources to provide excellent patient care.

The nurses' role in patient care has evolved with the use of technology to improve health care delivery.[1] Advancements in technology will continue to progress rapidly, and be the norm in health care rather than the exception. Hospitals are now high-tech environments, where electronic health records (EHR) have opened doors for emerging new technologies. These technologies, including EHRs, personal health records, clinical decision systems, computerized physician order entry, mobile technologies, wireless voice-over Internet phones (VOIP), radio frequency identification data tags (RFID), smart pumps, and telehealth, are examined in this article.

The Health Information Technology for Economic and Clinical Health (HITECH) Act, a component of the American Recovery and Reinvestment Act (ARRA) of 2009, encourages health care providers to become meaningful users of EHRs.[2,3] Beginning in 2015, reimbursement for health care services will be based on the adoption and use of the EHR.[2] Health care technology has also been identified as having a fundamental role in increased patient safety and cost-efficient care in the 2010 Institute of Medicine report titled "The Future of Nursing: Leading Change, Advancing Health."[4] Nursing is at the forefront and a driving force for the transformation of health care in the United States using health information technologies.[1]

Information and communication technology has become vital to patient care, allowing nurses to gather and share large amounts of information rapidly and efficiently.[5]

Disclosure statement: none.
Graduate Program, College of Health Sciences, School of Nursing, Walden University, 100 Washington Avenue, South Minneapolis, MN 55401, USA
E-mail address: debra.sullivan@waldenu.edu

0029-6465/15/$ – see front matter © 2015 Elsevier Inc. All rights reserved.

Nurses are known to be caring and, therefore, must use technology toward improving quality and safety of patient care.[6] Nurses have combined caring and technology to improve patient care as exemplified in an online survey, whereby 72% of registered nurses thought that medication safety had improved and 30% thought that information technology was a major contributor to those improvements.[7] In this ever-changing health care environment, caring and technology must go hand in hand to create a culture in nursing that embraces transformative technologies that are emerging every day.[6]

MEANINGFUL USE

The definition of *meaningful use* includes the use of certified EHRs to improve quality, safety, efficiency and reduce health disparities.[8] The information targeted by meaningful use is patient demographics, vital signs, charge changes, medication list, allergy list, current and active diagnosis, and smoking status.[9] Financial incentives to early adopters and the promise of future penalties for noncompliance from the Centers for Medicare and Medicaid Services to health care providers and organizations in the United States have accelerated the meaningful use program compliance[10] as described in the HITECH act of 2009.[2] Health care organizations and providers must be certified in health information technology (IT) and meet several criteria to receive the incentives.[10] The core objectives of the regulations involve providing patients and their primary care providers with information from the EHR, electronic ordering of prescriptions, evaluating drug interactions, tracking institutional compliance and quality improvement, and protecting the privacy and security of the EHR (**Table 1**).[9]

In a 2014 systematic review of 236 articles looking at health IT with a focus on meaningful use found the following summary points[10]:

1. Evaluation studies of health IT are increasing.[10]
2. Most evaluations focus on clinical decision support and computerized order entry.[10]
3. Most studies report positive effects on quality, safety, and efficiency.[10]
4. There is not enough information published to determine why some health IT implementation programs are successful and some are not.[10]
5. The most important improvement needed in health IT is increased measurement, analysis, and reporting of effects.[10]

ELECTRONIC HEALTH RECORDS

An EHR is an electronic or digital version of the traditional patient chart.[9] EHRs make information available instantly and securely through authorized users and are shared with other providers across various organizations.[9] EHRs can include patient demographics, medical history, diagnosis, medication, treatment plans, immunization

Table 1 Stages of meaningful use		
Stage 1: 2011–2012	**Stage 2: 2014**	**Stage 3: 2015**
Meaningful use criteria focus on: data capture and sharing	Meaningful use criteria focus on: advanced clinical processes	Meaningful use criteria focus on: improved outcomes

Adapted from HealthIT.gov. Meaningful use definition & objectives. Available at: https://www.healthit.gov/providers-professionals/meaningful-use-definition-objectives. Accessed May 13, 2015.

dates, allergies, radiology images and reports, and test results.[9] Tools that providers can use to make clinical-based decisions can be accessed from the EHR.[9] EHRs streamline health care provider work flow.[11]

Unfortunately, a 2012 survey reported that only 44% of hospitals used at least a basic EHR system.[11] Also reported was that 42.2% met the meaningful use stage 1 criteria, with 5.1% meeting stage 2 criteria.[11] Large urban hospitals had more EHRs in place than rural and nonteaching hospitals.[11] Giving patients access to their own clinical data is part of stage 2 criteria and many have a portal feature that allows patients to view test results, request a medication refill, and request appointments.[11] However, there are still barriers to allowing full access to patients because of security risks.[11] Another issue is that hospital systems are still not at the point of exchanging information between organizations and public health departments, mostly because of rural areas not having broadband Internet service.[11] In summary, the financial incentives for ARRA/HITECH are working as intended, but more technology infrastructure is needed before smaller and rural hospitals will be able to meet the stage 2 meaningful use criteria.[11]

There are benefits to EHRs as they can leverage other technologies and incorporate other digital processes. In addition, EHRs can transform delivery of health care and compensation.[12] Health care quality and convenience is improved for both the provider and patients with quick and remote access to patient records.[12] A national survey of doctors reported that EHRs saved time by efficient record retrieval and enhanced data confidentiality.[12] Large hospitals saved from $37 million to $59 million over 5 years, in addition to the incentive payments.[12] Savings are found in being able to track patients' use of hospital resources, such as equipment, supplies, testing, medication, and staff, which were sometimes lost in paper systems.[13] EHRs reduce errors, improve patient safety, and support better patient outcomes by providing alerts and reminders, analysis of information, and enabling evidence-based care at the point of care.[12]

Of course, there are issues related to EHRs. With the many different vendors of EHRs and security risks of sharing information, it is very difficult to share information between organizations, patients, and providers.[13] Cost is constraining; not only are there costs associated with the purchase of hardware and software but implementation expenditures can also be considerable for setup, maintenance, training IT support, and system updates.[13] Productivity can decrease for several weeks or more because of implementation.[13] The biggest issue is autofill or copy-and-paste functions that are meant to save time but can cause documentation errors, thereby putting patient safety at risk.[13]

There are advantages and disadvantages to EHRs, but they are here to stay. Being cognizant of the shortcomings and planning will help make purchase decisions, costs, implementation, and maintenance less painful.[13] Notably there have not been any recent studies that have found a consistent relationship between the use of EHRs and improved hospital performance.[14] In one randomized control study of 325 hospitals, there was no association between EHR adoption and the outcomes examined: acute myocardial infarction outcomes, risk-adjusted 30-day mortality, average length of stay, and average payment per discharge.[14] Clinical outcomes, such as improved quality and reduced medical errors, at the patient level have been studied with positive results.[15] Overall, experts agree that EHRs can benefit patients and society when widely adopted and used meaningfully.[15]

CLINICAL DECISION SYSTEMS

Clinical decision systems (CDS) are electronic systems that use individual patient information to generate patient-specific practice guidelines. CDSs can offer the health care provider recommendations to consider for patient care.[16] Classic CDSs include alerts, alarms, reminders, order sets, dashboards with performance feedback, drug-dose calculations, and information buttons.[16] Examples of CDSs are *UpToDate*, *Epocrates*, and *ClinicalKey*.[16]

CDS tools, such as physician reminders, have led to increased adherence to evidence-based practice and practice guidelines.[15] An example would be a physician reminder to order influenza and pneumococcal vaccinations. These types of reminders have increased adherence rates from 0% to 35% to 50% in hospitalized patients.[15,17] In another similar study in an outpatient setting among patients with rheumatoid patients, influenza vaccinations increased from 47% to 65% and pneumococcal vaccinations increased from 19% to 41% of patients.[15,18] Comparable results have been found in other studies whereby vaccination rates improved with computerized reminders.[15,19,20] In a 2012 systematic review of 160 articles, it was found that CDSs demonstrated efficacy across diverse settings.[16] CDSs were shown to have positive results related to prescribing treatments, facilitating preventive care services, and ordering clinical studies. More research is needed to gain a better understanding of what information is needed and should be delivered as well as a critical examination of unintended consequences of CDS.[16]

COMPUTERIZED PROVIDER ORDER ENTRY

Computerized Provider (Physician) Order Entry (CPOE) is a system whereby physicians or providers directly enter orders into a computer system, which then transmits the information to the appropriate department.[21] Historically with handwritten orders, it was found that medication errors occurred 90% of the time during the ordering or transcribing stage of writing orders.[21] CPOE eliminates the transcribing stage and assists the provider with ordering information, thus, has the potential to reduce errors.[21] For example, the physician enters a medication order into the CPOE system where dosage recommendations are reviewed; the order is then transmitted to the pharmacy where a patient medication administration record (MAR) is produced.[21] The MAR guides the pharmacist to provide the correct medication for the patient and the nurse on what medication to deliver to the patient. Many times CPOEs and paired with CDS systems as they complement each other.[21]

CPOE has been associated with a 55% reduction in serious medication errors.[15,22] Another study found that in an outpatient setting CPOE resulted in a reduction of errors from 18.2% down to 8.2%.[15,23,24] On the other hand, there have been studies that found an increase in medication errors associated with CPOE caused by poorly designed systems, lack of training, dense pull-down menus, or lack of integration.[15,25] In a 2014 systematic review of 19 studies that addressed CPOE and medication errors, CPOE was associated with more than 50% decline in the rate of injuries to patients caused by medication errors in hospital settings.[22] CPOE has the potential to benefit public health.[22]

BAR CODE MEDICATION ADMINISTRATION

When a health care provider uses an IT system to administer medication, it will interface with an EHR and usually a CPOE. By scanning the bar code on the medication and the patients' wrist band, the medication administration will be automatically documented into the MAR and can improve patient safety by verifying the correct medication is given in the right dose, at the right time, and to the correct patients.[26] There have been some problems with the implementation with nurse work-arounds, such as bypassing the scanning technology.[26] A quasi-experimental study was conducted of observing medication administrations over 9 months before and after implementing a bar code MAR system.[26] In the study, 14,041 medication administrations were observed; between the 2 groups, there was a 41.4% reduction in timing errors.[26] This study supports the use of bar-code technology as it improves safety by reducing medication and transcribing errors.[26]

PERSONAL HEALTH RECORD OR PATIENT PORTALS

A patient health record is also known as a patient portal and is defined as a secure on-line Web site that gives patients convenient 24-hour access to personal health information from anywhere with an Internet connection.[27] Using a secure username and password, patients can view health information, such as recent doctor visits, discharge summaries, medications, allergies, immunizations, and laboratory results.[27] Patient portals can also be used to schedule office visits, request medication refills, e-mail to ask questions, make payments, and view educational materials.[11,27]

The features of the patient portal benefit both patients and health care teams.[27] Portals are user friendly and are designed to alleviate the tension and frustration caused when patients are unable to speak with their clinician.[27] The portal allows for communication with patients without having to interrupt a busy clinic day to take phone calls. Patient portals are vehicles for meeting the meaningful use criteria by enabling secure messaging with health care providers and giving patients access to their personal health records.[28] Access to the portal is available 24 hours a day, 7 days a week through a secured HIPAA (Health Insurance Portability and Accountability Act)–compliant Web site.[29] Secure messaging with clinicians is one of the major highlights of patient portals. Clinicians have found great success in secure messaging and report an increase in efficiency, productivity, and a decrease in phone calls and mailing costs.[30]

Advocates of patient portals cite potential benefits with patient satisfaction, operational efficiency, and even clinical outcomes.[27] However, there is limited evidence to support these claims; therefore, more research is needed. One study looked at type 2 diabetic patients and the use of patient portals.[31] The conclusion was that secure messaging through the patient portal facilitated access to care, enhanced the quality of office visits, and increased patient satisfaction and clinical outcomes for diabetic patients.[31] As mentioned previously, there are still barriers to allowing full access to patient portals because of security risks.[11] Another issue is that hospital systems and patient accessibility are not at the point of easy access because of rural areas not having broadband Internet service.[11]

MOBILE TECHNOLOGY

Nurses are mobile, and they care for multiple patients; therefore, mobile technology is especially important for nurses.[32] The need for mobile tools can reduce errors and redundancy allowing the nurse to be at the patients' side more, instead of having to run to the nurses' station to gather information or communicate.[32] Mobile charting makes it easier to perform electronic charting and can save time and increase efficiency. As we use more and more point-of-care technologies, the need for mobile devices that can provide easy access to information is paramount. Some of the tools being used are electronic handoffs, task alerts, documentation of hourly rounding with the use of wireless tracking, the use of electronic medication records with built-in safety alerts, and wireless synchronized vital sign collection. A point-of-care technology scenario would look like this: A wireless glucometer synchronizes with a wireless network; the technician enters the blood sugar level to a point-of-care glucometer that automatically sends it to the patient's EHR; if the results are abnormal, the nurse receives an alert immediately on a mobile device.

The use of EHR requires that nurses have easy access to computers. Because of limited computer access and stationary computers located at nursing stations, nurses have tended to batch chart, saving charting responsibilities until they had a stopping point to catch up on charting.[33] The use of roving computers and other mobile charting devices allows the nurse to chart in real time and to gather current information about patients. A 2013 survey of 1000 nurses from across the United States asked about the reality of how technology at the bedside has improved patient care.[34] The results showed that 56.1% still have computers at the nurses' station; 53.5% have roving computers; and 31% have computers in each room. A newer technology, such as a tablet, is rarely (9.6%) used for charting even though 46% of the nurses own a personal tablet.[34]

In 2012 motion study of hospital nurses, it was found that nurses spent about the same amount of time charting with or without EHRs or computerized nursing notes.[35] Despite this, in a 2014 survey of hospital nurses,[33] nurses reported that they thought that electronic charting took more time than paper charting. Some of the reasons cited in the 2014 nurse study as disadvantages of mobile charting included too few devices; a lack of comfort, competence, or confidence in electronic documentation; and ineffective documentation.[33] Some advantages cited included time saving, increased time at bedside, improved interdisciplinary communication, and increased accuracy.[33] The information found illustrates how there is a need to increase the number of easily accessible mobile charting devices and point-of-care technologies.[33,34]

Mobile Wireless Voice-Over-Internet Protocol Phones

Traditional nurse call systems provide patients with a call button located at the bedside to push for help. The button signals a light at the nurses' station, and someone at the nurses' station responds to the patient initiating the call. That same person then pages the nurse over an intercom or to a pocket pager. This system prolongs the nurse response to the patients' needs, when nurses need to be easily reachable and responsive. Nurses can be more accessible with the use of mobile wireless VOIP phone systems.[32] These systems can notify the nurse of the room number, call priority, and the patient's name as well as allowing the nurse to respond.[36] Many of the phone systems have software that can be set to alert the nurse when preset physiologic parameters are breached, for example, in monitored vital signs or electrocardiogram rhythms. Some systems can track the nurse's location. Nurses have complained that the calls disrupt patient care while they are caring for other patients, but some systems will allow the call to roll over to another nurse based on their location to the patient.[36] According to the Cleveland Clinic, their VOIP system improves efficiency in communication between staff and patients and decreases noise.[32]

Radio Frequency Identification

Traditionally bar-code patient management systems identify patients using wristbands and can identify equipment and supplies using tags. Bar-code readers have worked nicely for medication administration. The nurse scans the patient's wristband with a bar code reader linked to an EHR and then scans the medication. The EHR medication administration software will confirm if this is the correct medication for this patient. Bar codes are fine when you have a line of sight needed to scan the barcode but do not help if items or people are lost. Another technology used more recently in hospitals is RFID tags. RFID tags use an electromagnetic or electrostatic connection in the radio frequency portion of the electromagnetic spectrum to distinctively identify an article, animal, or person.[37] There are 3 components needed for an RFID system to work: tags, readers, and antenna.[37] The RFID tags can be passive, which means they only communicate with the reader when they are sitting in range of the reader.[37] Passive RFID tags are mainly used for patient identification and medication administration.[37] The second category is battery-assisted passive RFID tags whereby the tag is powered by a battery but not used for communication purposes and only used to record sensor readings when not in use.[38] RFID tags can also be active, which means they can power integrated circuits and broadcast a signal to a reader, which can be wired or wireless networks.[37] Active RFID tags are used for tracking purposes.

These tags track at-risk patients, such as newborns in the nursery and wandering patients with Alzheimer disease.[32] They are also used to track nurses' movement and time in order to study traffic flow and time spent in patient care by shift, day of the week, and month.[39] They can work in conjunction with wireless phone systems to locate the nearest nurse. Hospitals are using both RFID and bar-code tags together as a fail-safe mechanism in case the RFID becomes unreadable.[39] In a systematic review of recent studies on RFIDs, they were found to improve patient safety, patient tracking and verification, tracking surgical items, operational efficiency (tracking equipment), and clinical errors (improve work flow of doctors, nurses, and caregivers).[37] Disadvantages included the high cost of complicated systems.[37] Even with the high cost of these systems, the advantages outweigh the disadvantages. Ultimately, RFID systems are cost-effective when you consider the improved quality of health care.[37]

Security is always an issue with wireless communication, and RFID tag security is no exception. The HIPAA governs and protects the security of patients' medical information, and RFID tags could reveal personal and private information. A breach in privacy is a serious concern. There are 4 ways security can be breached: interception (identity theft), interruption (degrading system performance), modification (injecting false data on the tags), and fabrication (duplicating valid tags or readers).[38] Physical security and limiting access can help prevent attacks to these systems. Coupling RFID with bar coding can be a check on patient identification. Programming the tags to transmit a short distance is another way to avoid this problem.[38] Using middleware systems that retrieve RFID data using security protocols to avoid privacy concerns is also being used.[37] Ongoing research must be done to avoid security issues.

Electronic Patient Tracking Boards

Areas of the hospital where high numbers of patients are managed for short periods, such as emergency departments (ED) and surgical areas, have traditionally used dry-erase whiteboards to track patients' status. Seen recently is the use of electronic whiteboards or electronic patient tracking boards that can integrate whiteboard information with the EHR.[40] They can broadcast information to multiple whiteboards, save information for later use, and improve communication. Electronic whiteboards can offer a quick status update of patients' current activity and streamline communication and coordination of patient care.[32] Because of the current technology, one can find these boards on many inpatient units, not just the ED or surgery.[32] Patient flow can be monitored by tracking patients, equipment, or staff members with RFID tags, which is transmitted and displayed in real time on electronic tracking boards.[41] Real-time location systems are also used for electronic patient tracking and reporting patient location, times, characteristics, and status, sometimes overlaid with a floor plan of a unit.[41] These systems communicate with EHRs, which provides information for areas besides nursing, such as bed management, patient admissions, and procedures.[41]

In a literature review of 21 studies on electronic whiteboards, it was found that there were positive and negative concerns for the work flow of EDs.[42] One of the problems cited was accuracy of the board's information. Rasmussen[42] also found that the board moves from being a clinician's tool to an administrative tool.[42] Positive findings were in patient satisfaction, length of stay, and financial and administrative aspects.[42] In a single study by Hertzum and Simonsen,[40] it was found that nurses were able to spend more time with their patients and less time at the control desk. Physicians did not report spending more time with patients.[40]

Use of electronic patient tracking is low at this time but growing.[41] ED and surgery department use is most common. Half of all patients go through the ED, and efficient placement of those going out to the hospital is essential. Surgery has the highest revenue, which makes efficient throughput and patient management crucial for financial health.[41] The investment return on these systems is not well studied, but there is a significant capital expenditure needed for these systems.[41] Overall, studies have shown the following among the many benefits of electronic patient tracking: decreased length of stay, improved utilization of resources, saved time for nurses, faster revenue generation, decreased paper costs, improved staff morale, better record keeping, and decreased liability.[41]

Smart Pumps

Historically, in the hospital setting, the administration of intravenous (IV) fluids was first administered with a drip rate calculated as drops per minute followed by infusion pumps, which have been around for about 40 years.[43] IV fluid administration carries a high risk for adverse drug events leading to the need for safety features on simple infusion pumps, which have evolved to smart pumps.[43] Smart pumps have software programs built into them to help prevent drug errors and include a drug library that has predefined parameters.[43] Drug libraries include tailored preloaded lists to a specific facility and patient care area.[44] The design is to ensure administration of appropriate dosing for a specific drug and, therefore, reduce medication miscalculations and errors.[43] There are hard limits, which are restrictive and do not allow the nurse to override, and soft limits that are not restrictive.[43] They also record all of the events for quality improvement.

Smart pumps do not eliminate the need for vigilant medication administration and the use of the 5 rights: right dose, right time, right drug, right patient, and right route. Nurses still need to assess the patients' vital signs and the IV site for phlebitis, infiltration, or extravasation. Despite the advanced technology of smart pumps, there continues to be programming and administrative errors.[44] The software relies on the accuracy of the programmed data entered into the smart pump.[45] There have been cases reported by the Food and Drug Administration (FDA) whereby the smart pump was programmed incorrectly by the pharmacist or administrator and another whereby the pump malfunctioned. Work-arounds are also a problem; this is when nurses use a nonstandard approach to solve a problem presented by technology and can put patients at risk.[45] An example of a work-around is bypassing the safety features on a smart pump.[45] A nurse can be found at fault for negligence if the smart pump is not used correctly and harms a patient.[46] The adoption rate of smart pumps has doubled since 2005 as other technologies have evolved, such as EHRs, computerized physician order entry, and bar-code medication administration.[43] If smart pumps are used at a facility, then they become the standard of care and must be used when available to enhance patient safety.[46]

Benefits of smart pumps include preventing medication errors, such as wrong rate, wrong dose, wrong pump setting, reduction of adverse drug event rates, cost-effectiveness, and practice improvement.[43] Other benefits include reduction of calculations, warnings, and alarm systems.[46] Negative effects include lower compliance of using smart pumps, overriding soft alerts, nonintercepted errors, or using the wrong drug library.[43] Smart pumps will continue to evolve and interface with other technologies in the health care setting.

Simulation

The use of high-fidelity simulation has become more acceptable in the hospital setting.[47] Hospital care has become more complex, and nurses make critical decisions associated with the care of more acute patients. Critical thinking, prioritization, and appropriate clinical decision making is a necessity in the nursing profession today.[48] Sound clinical judgment depends on being aware of what is happening during the episode and weighing how information, events, and your own actions will affect patient goals and objectives. Nurses must be able to not only gather information and anticipate patient needs but also make decisions in the best interest of their patients.[49] It is critical to prioritize the urgency of care, give care safely, detect changes in symptoms, voice concerns, and respond quickly.[49] As more of the current nursing workforce retires and newer nurses are employed within hospital systems, the educational challenges are providing opportunities to develop and/or enhance critical thinking and prioritization skills.

High-fidelity simulation provides an ideal environment to address and improve teamwork in high-acuity, stressful patient care scenarios and thereby mitigate the potential for human error. For better results in a specific area of training,[47] it is important to mirror the clinical environment as much as possible.[47] Providing an opportunity that allows multiple professional roles to interact will also help with interdisciplinary communication.[47]

Cost may be a barrier to simulation as simulators and the cost to create the environment is very expensive. There is an increasing number of simulated virtual world and simulation applications that could be an adjunct to live simulation. Employees could decrease training time by preparing for live simulation using these types of adjuncts.[47] Major health care institutions may consider offering simulation aimed at higher levels appropriate for senior staff related more to clinical judgment, clinical management, and organizational issues.[47]

TELEHEALTH AND MOBILE HEALTH

Advancements in technology have allowed for services, such as telehealth, which bring new ways to educate and access patients.[50] In the following discussion, telehealth, mobile health (mHealth), and remote monitoring are discussed. Telehealth is a means to communicate electronically between patients and health care providers, allowing for real-time health care.[50] mHealth uses mobile devices to communicate with health care providers and to acquire information and self-help–type applications. Remote monitoring monitors environmental changes that can offer seniors independence.

Telehealth

Telehealth offers low-cost health care with mobile devices, such as laptops, tablets, and smartphones.[32] These devices can replace expensive face-to-face visits with the use of videoconference capabilities.[32] There is a wide variety of services offered, including video consultation, asynchronous transfer of medical images, and the use of remote monitoring devices.[51] They can transmit vital signs and medical history to receive remote diagnosis and monitoring.[32] Medicare has approved payment for services provided for home health care services, which includes telehealth services.[51–54] The American Telemedicine Association defines telehealth as the delivery of remote health care using technology but not necessarily clinical services.[55] Telemedicine is differentiated as remote health care using technology that *does* offer clinical services.[55]

The use of telehealth is especially helpful for rural areas, the aging, and those with chronic illness[52] The Veterans Administration reported that with telehealth services, mental health and counseling services, and those with chronic health conditions had a long-term effect of reduced hospital use.[52] The use of telehealth in nursing homes has also dramatically reduced face-to-face consultation.[52]

Remote Monitoring

Remote monitoring is another technology that improves quality of life. With the use of sensors, motion detectors, and wireless technology, changes in behavior and activity are recorded and transmitted to the health care provider.[52] These sensors are considered passive sensors whereby information is monitored around the clock, such as vital signs, motion, falls, or even temperature of a stove top.[52] For the most part, these monitoring devices offer the senior autonomy, but sometimes false alerts can be frustrating to patients and the health care provider.[52] Active monitoring occurs when the senior interacts with the technology to record information, such as vital signs or blood glucose level, and then transmits the information to a health care provider. These systems can remind the senior of tasks like medication reminders or to keep their legs elevated.

The use of remote monitoring allows seniors to age in place and gives them the opportunity to stay in familiar settings where they are comfortable. This technology enhances quality of life, increases autonomy, and provides emotional benefits.[52] Telehealth technologies in general will continue to advance to offer more services as technology continues to advance.

Mobile Health

Mobile health, also referred to as mHealth, is the use of mobile devices to download medical information and to communicate with health care providers.[52] mHealth is one of the top 10 consumer mobile applications (apps) for 2012.[32] Cell phones are providing Latino and African American communities and illegal aliens a way for nurses to reach out with health tips and reminders concerning maternal health, human immunodeficiency virus/AIDS, and drug addiction.[32] Apple iPhone (Apple Inc, Cupertino, CA) has more than 213 apps that are related to chronic disease and even more for maternal health, with more than 5000 apps that are health related.[52] For example, a medication reminder app will let patients know when it is time to take medicine. A smoking cessation app will send text messages requesting support during cravings or withdrawal symptoms.[56]

In a systematic review of 75 randomized control trials of mHealth health care studies, 26 interventions to increase healthy behaviors and 49 targeted disease management interventions were reviewed.[56] Results of the review offered mixed evidence about the benefits of the interventions.[56] Smoking cessation support more than doubled verified smoking cessation.[56] However, diabetes control, medication reminders, and diet and exercise apps offered borderline clinical significance.[56] More research is needed to establish the benefits of mHealth to optimize health intervention apps.

Electronic Intensive Care Unit

Another telehealth service is the electronic intensive care unit (eICU). Intensive care units in remote areas can be monitored at a central location where intensivist physicians staff an eICU.[32] Through a constant link, small microphones, cameras, and vital information, such as heart rate, blood pressure, medications, and test results, are transmitted to the central location in real time. If a change occurs, the eICU nurses or physicians can activate a 2-way visual and audio link for immediate consultation.[32]

The costs of implementation, operation, and staffing were a major concern for hospitals adopting an eICU.[57] Responses from 10 eICUs lauded the eICU software and liked the immediate response to emergencies.[57] In a study of intensive care units in rural and urban regions in a developing country found that eICU was associated with significant improvement in mortality.[58] Contrary to other results of eICU research, 2 large eICU programs studied the effectiveness of selected parameters and did not find statistical significance.[59] The parameters looked at were rate of falls, mortalities, incidence of code blues, and length of stay before and after eICU implementation.[59] The outcome showed no statistically significant differences between before and after implementation. It is estimated that only 9% of intensive care unit beds in the United States use eICU; however, there are few studies that have looked at the effectiveness.[57]

SUMMARY

The HITECH Act of 2009 encourages health care providers to become meaningful users of EHRs.[2,5] Beginning in 2015, reimbursement for health care services will be based on the adoption and use of the EHR.[2,5] Meaningful use includes the use of certified EHRs to improve quality, safety, and efficiency and reduce health disparities.[8] Unfortunately, a 2012 survey reported that only 44% of hospitals used at least a basic EHR system.

EHRs can leverage other technologies and incorporate other digital processes. In addition, EHRs can transform the way health care is delivered and compensated.[12] Health care quality and convenience is improved for both the provider and patients with quick and remote access to patient records.[12] Experts agree that EHRs can benefit patients and society when widely adopted and used meaningfully.[15]

Examples of technology that complement EHRs are CDS and CPOE; when used with bar-code scanning technology, they can greatly reduce medication errors, with a 55% reduction in serious medication errors.[15,22] Patient health records, also known as patient portals, are vehicles for meeting the meaningful use criteria by enabling secure messaging with health care providers and giving patients access to their personal health records.[28]

The need for mobile tools can reduce errors and redundancy allowing the nurse to be at the patients' side more instead of having to run to the nurses' station to gather information or communicate.[32] Examples of mobile technology include VOIP phone systems that allow nurses to be at the bedside more and RFID tags that can track nurses, patients, equipment, medication, and supplies. Mobile charting makes it easier to perform electronic charting and can save time and increase efficiency. Electronic patient tracking boards can offer a quick status update of patients' current activity and streamline communication and coordination of patient care.[32] Smart pumps can prevent medication errors, such as wrong rate, wrong dose and pump setting, as well as reducing adverse drug event rates, while being cost-effective.[43] High-fidelity simulations provide an ideal environment to address and improve teamwork in high-acuity, stressful patient care scenarios and thereby mitigate the potential for human error. Advancements in technology have allowed for services, such as telehealth, which bring new ways to educate and access patients.[50] The use of sensors, motion detectors, and wireless technology can monitor changes in behavior and activity. This information is recorded and transmitted to the health care provider.[52]

Nurses are caring and, therefore, must use technology to complement patient care.[6] In this ever-changing health care environment, caring and technology must go hand in hand to create a culture in nursing that embraces transformative technologies that are emerging every day.[6]

REFERENCES

1. Carrington JM, Tiase VL. Nursing informatics year in review. Nurs Adm Q 2013; 37(2):136–43.
2. H.R. 1—111th Congress: American Recovery and Reinvestment Act. 2009. Gov-Track.us (database of federal legislation). [Context Link]. Available at: http://www.govtrack.us/congress/bills/111/hr1. Accessed May 30, 2015.
3. Institute of Medicine. The future of nursing: leading change, advancing health. [Context Link]. 2010. Available at: http://books.nap.edu/openbook.php?record_id=12956&page=R1. Accessed December 9, 2012.
4. Fujino Y, Kawamoto R. Effect of information and communication technology of nursing performance. Comput Inform Nurs 2013;31(5):244–50.
5. Ball MJ, Douglas JC, Hinton WP, et al. Nursing informatics: where technology and caring meet. London; Dordrecht (Netherlands); Heidelberg (Germany); New York: Springer; 2011.
6. Weier S. RNs cite IT as 'major contributor' to medication safety improvements. Burlington (MA): iHealth-Beat; 2005. Available at: www.ihealthbeat.org.
7. Hogan S, Kisam S. Measuring meaningful use. Health Aff 2010;29(4):600–6.
8. Jones S, Rudin R, Perry T, et al. Health information technology: an updated systematic review with a focus on meaningful use [serial online]. Ann Intern Med 2014;160(1):48–54.
9. HealthIT.gov. What is an electronic health record (EHR)? Available at: http://www.healthit.gov/providers-professionals/faqs/what-electronic-health-record-ehr. Accessed June 8, 2015.
10. Rabius V, Karam-Hage M, Blalock JA, et al. "Meaningful use" provides a meaningful opportunity. Cancer 2013;120(4):464–8.
11. DesRoches CM, Dustin C, Furukawa MF, et al. Adoption of electronic health records grows rapidly, but fewer than half of US hospital had at least a ASIC in 2012. Health Aff 2013;32(8):1478–85.
12. HealthIT.gov. Benefits of electronic health records (EHRs). Available at: http://www.healthit.gov/providers-professionals/benefits-electronic-health-records-ehrs. Accessed June 8, 2015.
13. Palma G. Electronic health records: the good, the bad and the ugly. Beckers Health IT & CIO Review. 2013. Available at: http://www.beckershospitalreview.com/healthcare-information-technology/electronic-health-records-the-good-the-bad-and-the-ugly.html. Accessed June 8, 2015.
14. Adler-Milstein J, Scott K, Jha AK. Leveraging EHRs to improve hospital performance: the role of management. Am J Manag Care 2014;20(11 Spec No.17): SP511–29.
15. Menachemi N, Ollum TH. Benefits and drawbacks of electronic health record systems. Risk Manag Healthc Policy 2011;4:47–55.
16. Bright T, Wong A, Lobach D, et al. Effect of clinical decision-support systems: a systematic review [serial online]. Ann Intern Med 2012;157(1):29–43.
17. Dexter PR, Perkins S, Overhage JM, et al. A computerized reminder system to increase the use of preventive care for hospitalized patients. N Engl J Med 2001;345(13):965–70.

18. Ledwich LJ, Harrington TM, Ayoub WT, et al. Improved influenza and pneumo-coccal vaccination in rheumatology patients taking immunosuppressants using an electronic health record best practice alert. Arthritis Rheum 2009;61(11): 1505–10.

19. McDonald CJ, Hui SL, Tierney WM. Effects of computer reminders for influenza vacci-nation on morbidity during influenza epidemics. MD Comput 1992;9(5):304–12.

20. Tierney WM, Hui SL, McDonald CJ. Delayed feedback of physician performance versus immediate reminders to perform preventive care. Effects on physician compliance. Med Care 1986;24(8):659–66.

21. Agency for Healthcare Research and Quality (AHRQ). Computerized provider or-der entry. Available at: http://psnet.ahrq.gov/primer.aspx?primerID=6. Accessed June 8, 2015.

22. Nuckols TK, Smith-Spangler C, Morton SC, et al. The effectiveness of computer-ized order entry at reducing preventable adverse drug events and medication er-rors in hospital settings: a systematic review and meta-analysis. Syst Rev 2014; 3(56):1–12.

23. Bates DW, Leape LL, Cullen DJ, et al. Effect of computerized physician order en-try and a team intervention on prevention of serious medication errors. JAMA 1998;280(15):1311–6.

24. Devine EB, Hansen RN, Wilson-Norton JL, et al. The impact of computerized pro-vider order entry on medication errors in a multispecialty group practice. J Am Med Inform Assoc 2010;17(1):78–84.

25. Campbell EM, Sittig DF, Ash JS, et al. Types of unintended consequences related to computerized provider order entry. J Am Med Inform Assoc 2006;13(5): 547–56.

26. Poon EG, Keohane CA, Yoon CS, et al. Effect of bar-code technology on the safety of medication administration. N Engl J Med 2010;362(18):1698–707. Avail-able at: http://search.proquest.com/docview/223925866?accountid=14872.

27. HealthIT.gov. What is a patient portal? Available at: http://www.healthit.gov/providers-professionals/faqs/what-patient-portal. Accessed May 13, 2015.

28. Otte-Trojel T, Bont A, Van de Klundert J, et al. Characteristics of patient portals developed in the context of health information exchanges: early policy effects of incentives in meaningful use program in the United States. J Med Internet Res 2014;16(11):e258.

29. Louiselle P. Utilizing patient portal functionality within an EMR system. J Med Pract Manage 2012;28(3):183–6.

30. Peck AD. Optimize your patient portal: the key to persuading patient to use your portal is developing strategy based on communication and eduction, physicians say. Med Econ 2014;91(17):48–50, 52.

31. Wade-Vunturo AE, Mayberry LS, Osborn CY. Secure messaging and diabetes management: experiences and perspective of patient portal users. J Am Med Inform Assoc 2013;20(3):519–25.

32. Minority Nurse Staff. Charts are going mobile. New York: Springer; 2013. Avail-able at: http://minoritynurse.com/charts-are-going-mobile/. Accessed May 27, 2015.

33. Hirsch A. Technology management strategies for nurse leaders. Nurs Manag 2014;45:41–3.

34. Hader R. How connected are you? Nurs Manag 2013;44:19–23.

35. Yee T, Needleman J, Pearson M, et al. The influence of integrated electronic med-ical records and computerized nursing notes on nurses' time spent in documen-tation. Comput Inform Nurs 2012;30(6):287–92.

36. Unluturk MS, Ozcanhan MH, Dalkilic G. Improving communication among nurses and patients. Comput Methods Programs Biomed 2015;120:103–12.
37. Ajami S, Carter MW. The advantages and disadvantages of radio frequency identification (RFID) in health-care centers; approach in emergency room (ER). Pak J Med Sci 2013;29(Suppl 1):443–8.
38. Hawrylak P, Schimke N, Hale J, et al. Security risks associated with radio frequency identification in medical environments [serial online]. J Med Syst 2012; 36(6):3491–505.
39. Reeder S. Radio frequecncy identification device (RFID) and real time location systemes (RTLS) enhance nursing care delivery. 25th International Nursing Research Congress. Hong Kong, July 26, 2014.
40. Hertzum M, Simonsen J. Work-practice changes associated with an electronic emergency department whiteboard. Health Informatics J 2013;19(1):46–60.
41. Drazen E, Rhoads J. Using tracking tools to improve patient flow in hospitals: issue brief. Oakland (CA): California Healthcare Foundation; 2011. Available at: http://www.chcf.org/~/media/MEDIA%20LIBRARY%20Files/PDF/U/PDF%20Using PatientTrackingToolsInHospitals.pdf. Accessed May 27, 2015.
42. Rasmussen R. Electronic whiteboards in emergency medicine: a systematic review. In Proceedings of the 2nd ACM SIGHIT International Health Informatics Symposium. ACM; p. 483–92.
43. Ohashi K, Dalleur O, Dykes PC, et al. Benefits and risks of using smart pumps to reduce medication error rates: a systematic review. Drug Saf 2014;37(12):1011–20.
44. Cummings K, McGowan R. Smart infusion pumps are selectively intelligent. Nursing 2011;41(3):58–9.
45. Kirkbride G, Vermace B. Smart pumps: implications for nurse leaders. Nurs Adm Q 2011;34(2):110–8.
46. Harding AD. Intravenous smart pumps. J Infus Nurs 2013;36(3):191–4.
47. Arora S, Cox C, Savies S, et al. Towards the next frontier for simulation-based training: full hospital simulation across the entire patient pathway. Ann Surg 2013;00:1–7.
48. Kaddoura MA. New graduate nurses' perceptions of the effects of clinical simulation on their critical thinking, learning, and confidence. J Contin Educ Nurs 2010;41(1):506–16.
49. Fero LJ, Witsberger DM, Wesmiller SW, et al. Critical thinking ability of new graduate and experience nurses. J Adv Nurs 2009;65(1):139–48.
50. Monigle D, Mastrian K. Introduction to information, information science and information systems. In: Mcgonigle D, Mastrian K, editors. Nursing informatics and the foundation of knowledge. 2nd edition. UA: Jones & Barlett Learning; 2012. p. 22.
51. US Department of Health and Human Services. Evaluation and research studies for ORDI system of record. Washington, DC: Centers for Medicare & Medicaid Services; 2010.
52. Goldwater J, Harris Y. Using technology to enhance the aging experience: a market analysis of existing technologies. Ageing Int 2011;36:5–28.
53. US Department of Health and Human Services. Glossary of terms. Washington, DC: Assistant Secretary for Planning and Evaluation; 2010.
54. US Department of Health and Human Services. Medicare benefit policy manual. Washington, DC: Centers for Medicare & Medicaid Services; 2010.
55. What is telemedicine? American Telemedine Association. Available at: http://www.americantelemed.org/about-telemedicine/what-is-telemedicine#.VWaFPM_BzRY. Accessed May 27, 2015.

56. Free C, Phillips G, Galli L, et al. The effectiveness of mobile-health technology-based health behavior change or disease management interventions for health care consumers: a systematic review. PLoS Med 2013;10(1):e1001362.
57. Berenson RA, Grossman JM, November EA. Does telemonitoring of patients-the eICU-improve intensive care. Health Aff 2009;28(5):w937–47.
58. Gupta S, Dewan S, Kaushal A, et al. eICU reduces mortality in STEMI patients in resource limited areas. Glob Heart 2014;9(4):425–7.
59. Dhakal A, Dhakal B, Pathak LK, et al. eICU study: a proof of concept. IJUDH 2014;4(2):5.

Validation of the National Institutes of Health Patient-Reported Outcomes Measurement Information System Survey as a Quality-of-Life Instrument for Patients with Malignant Brain Tumors and Their Caregivers

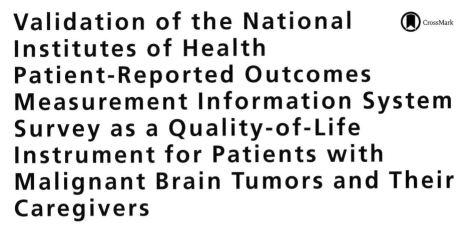

Melissa M. Romero, PhD, FNP-BC[a],*, Lisa Sue Flood, DNP[a],
Nanci K. Gasiewicz, DNP, RN, CNE[a], Richard Rovin, MD[b],
Samantha Conklin, MSN, FNP-BC[a]

KEYWORDS

• Quality of life • Malignant brain tumor • Caregiver • Pilot study • iPod touch device

KEY POINTS

• Quality-of-life issues are a major concern for individuals with malignant brain tumors and their caregivers.

• Quality-of-life assessments are challenging because of a lack of well-validated surveys and self-reporting difficulties that may occur in patients with malignant brain tumors.

• This pilot study used correlational methods to compare the National Institutes of Health Patient-Reported Outcomes Measurement Information System (NIH PROMIS) survey with 3 established and well-validated quality-of-life surveys in patients with malignant brain tumors and their caregivers.

• Results from the study provided some support for use of the NIH PROMIS as a quality-of-life measure in patients with malignant brain tumors and their caregivers.

Disclosures: None.
Funding: This work was supported by a faculty grant from Northern Michigan University (Grant number: 5-54867).
Conflicts of Interest: None of the authors have conflicts of interest to declare.
[a] School of Nursing, Northern Michigan University, 2131 New Science Facility, 1401 Presque Isle Avenue, Marquette, MI 49855, USA; [b] Marquette General Neurosurgery, UP Health System Marquette, 580 West College Avenue, Marquette, MI 49855, USA
* Corresponding author.
E-mail address: mromero@nmu.edu

INTRODUCTION

Approximately 70,000 new cases of primary brain tumors were diagnosed in the United States in 2014, with about 24,620 of those cases being malignant brain tumors.[1] The prognosis for individuals diagnosed with glioblastoma multiforme, an advanced form of malignant brain tumor, is dismal, with a median survival time of 12 to 14 months for patients who receive treatment and 3 months for patients who decline treatment.[2] Treatment options for patients with malignant brain tumors consist of surgery, radiation, and chemotherapy. The poor prognosis coupled with physical and mental impairments associated with malignant brain tumors and adverse treatment effects may negatively affect a person's quality of life. Depending on the location of the tumor, individuals may experience a variety of symptoms, including nausea, sleeplessness, visual defects, personality changes, headache, anorexia, aphasia, and seizures.[3]

Quality-of-life issues are a major concern for individuals with malignant brain tumors and their caregivers.[4–7] Caregivers of persons with malignant brain tumors are usually family members consisting of spouses or adult children. Researchers have indicated that providing care for a family member with a malignant brain tumor can lead to caregivers experiencing major life disruptions and subsequent reductions in quality of life consisting of increased symptoms of anxiety and depression, marital strain, psychosomatic symptoms, diminished social relationships, and physical health problems.[7] Weitzner and colleagues[7] found that caregivers with decreased mental health experienced reductions in their overall quality of life.

There is a need for reliable and valid quality-of-life questionnaires that are easy to use for both patients with malignant brain tumors and their caregivers.[4,5,8] Information from these surveys could provide nurses and other health care providers with knowledge about issues that affect quality of life so that specific interventions could be developed to enhance the lives of patients with malignant brain tumors and their caregivers. In a literature review that examined quality of life in patients with brain tumors, Liu and colleagues[5] acknowledged that quality-of-life assessments are challenging because of a lack of well-validated surveys and self-reporting difficulties that occur in this patient population as a result of functional and cognitive impairments. These investigators recommended validation of easy-to-use, quality-of-life questionnaires and continued exploration of factors that contribute to quality of life in patients with brain tumors, such as caregiver support.[5]

Other researchers have indicated that some patients with malignant brain tumors struggle to complete pen-and-paper surveys because of neurologic changes, medications, and treatment effects.[4,5] Using a computer-based quality-of-life instrument to monitor patients with brain tumors in an outpatient clinic setting, Erharter and colleagues[8] found that some patients needed supervision or proxy help to enter data. The investigators concluded that although practice implications related to patient and caregiver communication need to be further explored, immediate results from computer quality-of-life surveys could give health care providers important data needed for interventions.[8]

PURPOSE OF THE STUDY

The primary purpose of this pilot study was to validate components of the National Institutes of Health Patient-Reported Outcomes Measurement Information System (NIH PROMIS) survey as a quality-of-life instrument for patients with primary malignant brain tumors and their caregivers. The NIH PROMIS is a computer-adapted survey that was developed to measure patient-reported outcomes for individuals with a wide variety of chronic diseases and demographic characteristics. Before being used to measure quality of life in patients with primary malignant brain tumors and their caregivers in a health care setting, the NIH PROMIS survey must be validated by comparing it with other quality-of-life measures that have been validated in these same populations. This research aims to validate components of the NIH PROMIS survey by comparing it with 2 already established quality-of-life measures: the European Organization for Research and Treatment of Cancer (EORTC-30) questionnaire and the Caregiver Quality-of-Life Cancer (CQOLC) scale.

The secondary purpose of this study was to evaluate the use of the iPod Touch mobile device as a means to complete and submit the quality-of-life surveys. Symptoms experienced by patients with brain tumors can make self-reporting difficult. Consequently, a need exists for user-friendly, effective methods for persons with brain tumors and their caregivers to provide information about their quality of life. The iPod Touch is a hand-held, touch-screen device that has the potential to be a feasible and convenient way to collect quality-of-life data from the study population.

RESEARCH QUESTIONS

The following research questions were explored:

1. How do the quality-of-life scores of adult patients with malignant brain tumors on the NIH PROMIS survey compare with their results on the EORTC-30 survey?
2. How do the quality-of-life scores of caregivers of adult patients with malignant brains tumors on the NIH PROMIS survey compare with their results on the CQOLC survey?
3. Can adult patients with primary malignant brain tumors and their caregivers effectively use hand-held devices (iPod Touch) to complete quality-of-life surveys?

METHODS
Study Sample and Procedures

A descriptive, correlational design was used with a convenience sample of 10 patients diagnosed with primary malignant brain tumors and 10 of their caregivers (N = 20). A neurosurgeon and nursing faculty participated in a collaborative, interdisciplinary partnership for this study. Institutional Review Board approval was obtained from the hospital and university before the study. Ten patients with malignant brain tumors and their caregivers were recruited during the fall of 2011 and winter of 2012. Inclusion criteria consisted of the following items: (1) aged 18 years or older, (2) being able to read and speak English (quality-of-life surveys are language specific), (3) having a caregiver who agreed to participate in the study, and (4) having a confirmed tissue diagnosis of primary malignant brain tumor (eg, malignant glioma or oligodendroglioma, anaplastic astrocytoma, glioblastoma multiforme). Exclusion criteria included the following items: (1) inability to read and speak English, (2) having a diagnosis of benign primary brain tumor (eg, meningioma, pituitary adenoma), (3) having a diagnosis of metastatic brain tumor, (4) having a caregiver who declined participation in the study, and (5) being younger than 18 years of age. Participants were informed that after beginning the study, if a patient or their caregiver was unable or unwilling to participate, the other member of the pair could continue with the study if desired.

Participant Recruitment

Eligible patients and their caregivers were recruited for the study before scheduled outpatient neurosurgery clinic visits during the fall of 2011 and winter of 2012. Before the clinic visit, prospective participants were contacted via telephone by a neurosurgeon at the clinic who provided basic information about the study. After meeting with the neurosurgeon for the regular scheduled clinic visit, trained research assistants and a nursing faculty member provided detailed information to patient/caregiver dyads about the study background, objectives, patient protections, and procedures. After consent was obtained, participants received detailed instructions from the trained research assistants on use of the iPod Touch and quality-of-life survey applications. After receiving the instructions, each participant received a study packet containing a copy of the signed consent forms, a demographic survey, researcher contact information, and an iPod Touch device that had been preprogrammed with patient and caregiver random 6-digit identification numbers. The use of random 6-digit identification numbers ensured that the participants' data remained anonymous. The iPod Touch had a preloaded application (app) that contained the quality-of-life surveys used in the study. Research assistants helped with the setup of the devices before the start of the study.

Data Collection

Research assistants and a nursing faculty member assisted the patient/caregiver dyads with completion of the surveys using the iPod Touch device. Participants were asked to enter their identification number for data-tracking purposes before beginning the iPod Touch surveys. Next, the patient participants used the iPod Touch to complete the NIH PROMIS and EORTC-30 surveys. The caregiver participants then completed the NIH PROMIS and CQOLC surveys. Finally, after the surveys were completed, patient/caregiver dyads were asked to complete a pen-and-paper exit survey, which assessed the feasibility of using the iPod Touch and participants' thoughts and feelings about the individual surveys.

MEASURES
Demographic Information

A demographic form included questions about age, gender, and race; level of education; patient biopsy results; treatments (eg, surgery, chemotherapy, radiation); and date of the patient's tissue diagnosis. The demographic form also included questions about level of experience with computers and smartphones or similar devices.

Quality-of-Life Measures

The NIH PROMIS[9] survey was used to measure quality of life in caregivers and patients with malignant brain tumors. The NIH PROMIS comprises of a multitude of quality-of-life domains. For the purposes of the present study, the following 7 quality-of-life domains in patients with malignant brain tumors were selected: (1) Sleep Disturbance, (2) Sleep-Related Impairment, (3) Pain Behavior, (4) Pain Interference, (5) Social Activity, (6) Social Role, and (7) Physical Function. In caregivers, the following 6 domains were examined: (1) Sleep Disturbance, (2) Sleep Related-Impairment, (3) Social Activity, (4) Social Role, (5) Depression, and (6) Anxiety. Because the survey is designed to be adaptive, an algorithm is used to determine the number and content of survey items within domains, based on participants' responses to previous questions. Therefore, the number of items per domain may vary. Items within each domain are rated on a 5-point Likert scale ranging from 5 (not at all) to 1 (very much). For each domain, a score of 50 is considered average within the United States general population, with most individuals scoring between 40 and 60 and almost all individuals scoring between 30 and 70. Lower scores reflect lower levels of quality of life. Sample domain items include: (1) "Are you able to walk a block on flat ground?" (physical function), (2) "In the past 7 days I felt worried" (anxiety), and (3) "In the past 7 days I could not stop feeling sad" (depression). Cronbach α for the total score in this study was 0.903, and scores for the domains of Sleep (sleep disturbance/sleep related impairment), Pain (pain behavior/pain interference), and Social (social activity/social role) were 0.817, 0.955, and 0.938 respectively. The instrument demonstrates high internal consistency, reliability, and established validity in prior studies of patients with chronic pulmonary disease exacerbation, rheumatoid arthritis, congestive heart failure, depression, and back and leg pain.[9]

A modified version of the EORTC-30[10] survey was used to measure quality of life in patients with malignant brain tumors. The EORTC-30 is a 30-item cancer-related quality-of-life survey that contains 3 domains comprising multiple subscales. The Functional domain contains 5 subscales: (1) physical, (2) role, (3) cognitive, (4) social, and (5) emotional. The Symptom domain contains 9 subscales (fatigue, pain, nausea/vomiting, dyspnea, insomnia/sleep, appetite loss, constipation, diarrhea, and financial difficulty). Finally, the Global Health/Quality of Life domain contains 2 single-item symptom measures that use a numeric scale ranging from 1 (very poor) to 7 (excellent). Scores for the first 28 items are rated on a 4-point Likert scale ranging from 1 (not at all) to 4 (very much). For the purposes of the present study, 11 questions were selected from the following 4 subscales: (1) Insomnia/sleep function (2 items), (2) Physical function (5 items), (3) Social function (2 items), and (4) Pain (2 items). Sample subscale items include: (1) "During the past week: did pain interfere with your daily activities?" and (2) "Do you need help with eating, dressing, washing yourself or using the toilet?" Items were summed for a total score ranging from 11 to 44, with lower scores reflecting higher quality of life. Cronbach α for the total score in this study was 0.724, and scores for subscales of insomnia/sleep, pain, social function, and physical function were 0.825, 0.704, 0.615, and 0.751 respectively. The EORTC-30 instrument demonstrated high levels of internal consistency, reliability, and established validity in the original study.[10]

The CQOLC[7] survey was used to measure quality of life in caregivers of patients with malignant brain tumor. The CQOLC consists of 35 items, with lower scores reflecting higher levels of quality of life. Eight positively worded questions are reverse scored. The instrument comprises 6 quality-of-life domains: (1) Social Function, (2) Physical Function, (3) Psychological Function, (4) Financial, (5) Caregiver Burden, and (6) Family Function. For the purposes of this study, the authors examined responses from 8 questions that were selected from individual subscale items within the domains: (1) Social function (4 items), (2) Sleep (physical function; 1 item), (3) Depression (psychological function; 2 items), and (4) Anxiety (psychological function; 1 item). Sample items include: (1) "During the past 7 days, my daily life is imposed upon" (Caregiver Burden), (2) "During the past 7 days, I felt nervous" (Psychological Function), and (3) "I get support from my friends and family" (Social Function). Scores are rated on a 5-point Likert scale ranging from 0 (not at all) to 4 (very much). Items were summed for a total score ranging from 0 to 32. Cronbach α for the total score in the original study was 0.91 and the test-retest correlation coefficient was 0.91. The instrument was found to be a valid quality-of-life measure for caregivers of individuals with cancer.[7]

Exit Survey

A pen-and-paper exit survey was used to assess feasibility of using the iPod Touch, and participants' thoughts and feelings about the individual surveys. The exit survey consists of 11 questions and a request for written comments and suggestions. Sample items include: (1) "Overall, what did you think of the NIH PROMIS survey?," (2) "Which survey did you prefer?," and (3) "I liked taking these surveys using the iPod Touch." Responses were analyzed and evaluated by the research team.

DATA ANALYSIS

Data were entered and verified using SPSS-PC v.18.1. Descriptive statistics of mean, standard deviation (SD), and percentages were computed to describe the sample. Internal consistency of the NIH PROMIS and EORTC-30 instruments were examined using the Cronbach α coefficient, and to answer the research questions Pearson correlations were calculated to compare the NIH PROMIS instrument with the patient (EORTC-30) and caregiver (CQOLC) quality-of-life scores, respectively.

RESULTS
Sample Characteristics

All patients had been diagnosed with some form of malignant brain tumor. Four patients had been diagnosed with glioblastoma and 3 with astrocytoma, and 3 patients were unsure of their diagnosis but were aware that their brain tumor was malignant. At the time of the assessment, the average length of time since tissue diagnosis was 21.8 months (SD = 17). Patients' ages ranged from 33 to 76 years (mean = 59.6, SD = 14.9). The average age at the time of tissue diagnosis was 57.8 (SD = 14.9) years. Concerning treatment, all 10 patients had received a biopsy and 6 had previously undergone surgery for their brain tumor. Nine patients reported that they received chemotherapy and 7 that they received radiation therapy. Forty percent of the patients were female (n = 4), 6 were male (60%), and of these 9 were white and 1 was Native American. The caregivers in the present study were on average 57.9 (SD = 16.1) years old. Thirty percent of the caregivers were female (n = 3) and 7 were male (70%); 9 were white and 1 was Native American. All of the study participants had completed high school, 5 had completed some college courses, 4 had obtained a Bachelor's degree, and 4 had completed graduate school (**Table 1**).

With the exception of 1 patient/caregiver dyad, all participants owned a home computer, although only 3 participants (2 caregivers and 1 patient) owned an iPod Touch and/or smartphone. The majority (75%) of participants stated that they felt comfortable using a home computer, whereas 2 caregivers and 3 patients reported they were not comfortable using a computer. Before participating in the study, 85% of patient/caregiver dyads indicated that they were not experienced in using an iPod Touch or a smartphone.

Quality-of-Life Scores

The NIH PROMIS was used to measure quality of life in patients with malignant brain tumors and their caregivers. In patients, individual scores from items within all 7 domains (Sleep Disturbance, Sleep Related-Impairment, Pain Behavior, Pain Interference, Social Activity, Social Role, and Physical Function) ranged from 25 to 74 with

Table 1
Participants' characteristics

Characteristics	Total (N = 20)	Patients (n = 10)	Caregivers (n = 10)
Age, mean (SD), y	58.8 (15.5)	59.6 (14.9)	57.9 (16.1)
Sex			
Male	9	6	3
Female	11	4	7
Length of time since diagnosis, mean (SD), mo	—	21.8 (17.0)	—
Age at diagnosis, mean (SD), y	—	57.8 (14.9)	—
Race/ethnicity, n (%)			
White	18 (90)	9 (90)	9 (90)
Native American	2 (10)	1 (10)	1 (10)
Level of education, n (%)			
High school	20 (100)	10 (100)	10 (100)
Some college	5 (25)	3 (15)	2 (10)
Undergraduate degree	4 (20)	2 (10)	2 (10)
Graduate degree	4 (20)	1 (5)	3 (15)

a mean score of 48.5 (SD = 11.0). This result suggests that in general, quality of life was slightly below average because, as previously discussed, a score of 50 is considered to be average within the United States (**Table 2**).[9]

In caregivers, scores from items within all 6 domains (Sleep Disturbance, Sleep-Related Impairment, Social Activity, Social Role, Depression, and Anxiety) ranged from 32 to 71 with a mean score of 52.1 (SD = 7.7), which generally suggests that quality of life was slightly above average (see **Table 2**).

Quality of life in patients with malignant brain tumors was measured using 11 subscale items from the EORTC-30 survey: Insomnia/Sleep Function (2 items), Physical Function (5 items), Social Function (2 items), and Pain (2 items). Insomnia/Sleep Function, Physical Function, Social Function, and Pain scores ranged from 19 to 36 with a mean score of 24.7 (SD = 5.4), suggesting that overall quality of life was slightly below average (see **Table 2**).

In caregivers, quality of life was measured using 8 items from the CQOLC survey: Social Function (4 items), Sleep (1 item), Depression (2 items), and Anxiety (1 item). Social Function, Sleep, Depression, and Anxiety scores ranged from 4 to 22 with a mean score of 11.3 (SD = 6.2), suggesting a quality of life slightly above average (see **Table 2**).

Correlations

In patients with malignant brain tumors, the authors matched similar items across domains and subscales, and performed bivariate correlation analysis between NIH PROMIS domains of Sleep Disturbance, Sleep-Related Impairment, Pain Behavior, Pain Interference, Social Activity, Social Role, and Physical Function with items from the following EORTC-30 subscales: Insomnia/Sleep Function (2 items), Physical Function (5 items), Social Function (2 items), and Pain (2 items). The NIH PROMIS Sleep Disturbance domain correlated significantly with 1 of the

Table 2
Description of measures

Variable	Patients (n = 10)		Caregivers (n = 10)	
NIH PROMIS score[a]	48.5	(11.0)	52.1	(7.7)
NIH PROMIS domains[b]				
Sleep disturbance score	56.3	(10.7)	52.6	(8.8)
Sleep-related impairment score	53.2	(9.1)	51.2	(9.6)
Pain behavior score	45.4	(11.9)	—	—
Pain interference score	50.2	(13.3)	—	—
Social activity score	46.9	(9.6)	49.9	(7.6)
Social role score	42.6	(9.7)	48.2	(7.7)
Physical function score	44.6	(12.4)		
Depression score	—	—	54.3	(7.3)
Anxiety score	—	—	56.1	(5.4)
EORTC total score[c]	24.7	(5.4)	—	—
EORTC subscales and individual subscale items[d]				
Insomnia/sleep, total score[e]	6.0	(1.6)	—	—
Insomnia/sleep, item 1 score	3.0	(0.8)	—	—
Insomnia/sleep, item 2 score	3.0	(0.8)	—	—
Physical function total score[f]	8.9	(3.3)	—	—
Physical function, item 1 score	2.3	(1.1)	—	—
Physical function, item 2 score	2.1	(1.1)	—	—
Physical function, item 3 score	1.7	(1.1)	—	—
Physical function, item 4 score	1.4	(0.5)	—	—
Physical function, item 5 score	1.4	(0.5)	—	—
Social function total score[g]	3.8	(1.8)	—	—
Social function, item 1 score	1.8	(1.0)	—	—
Social function, item 2 score	2.0	(0.9)	—	—
Pain total score[h]	6.0	(1.6)	—	—
Pain, item 1 score	3.0	(0.8)	—	—
Pain, item 2 score	3.0	(0.8)	—	—
CQOLC total score[i]	11.3	(6.2)	—	—
CQOLC domains and subscale items[j]				
Social function domain total score[k]	4.1	(3.2)	—	—
Social function, item 1 score	1.1	(1.2)	—	—
Social function, item 2 score	1.2	(1.2)	—	—
Social function, item 3 score	1.0	(1.2)	—	—
Social function, item 4 score	0.8	(1.2)	—	—
Sleep subscale total score[l]	1.5	(1.6)	—	—
Depression subscale total score[m]	3.7	(2.8)	—	—
Depression, item 1 score	1.8	(1.5)	—	—
Depression, item 2 score	1.9	(1.4)	—	—
Anxiety subscale total score[n]	2.5	(1.2)	—	—

(continue on next page)

Values are expressed as mean (SD) unless otherwise indicated.
 [a] The range for possible scores is 30–70.
 [b] The range for possible scores is 30–70.
 [c] The range for possible scores is 11–44.
 [d] The range for possible individual item scores is 1–4.
 [e] The range for possible scores is 2–8.
 [f] The range for possible scores is 5–20.
 [g] The range for possible scores is 2–8.
 [h] The range for possible scores is 2–8.
 [i] The range for possible scores is 0–32.
 [j] The range for possible individual item scores is 0–4.
 [k] The range for possible scores is 0–16.
 [l] The range for possible scores is 0–4.
 [m] The range for possible scores is 0–8.
 [n] The range for possible scores is 0–4.

EORTC-30 Insomnia/Sleep Function items (P = .03). There were no significant associations between the NIH PROMIS Sleep-Related Impairment domain and Insomnia/Sleep items on the EORTC-30. NIH PROMIS Pain Behavior and Pain Interference domains did not correlate significantly with either of the EORTC-30 Pain items. NIH PROMIS Social Role and Social Functioning were not associated with either of the EORTC-30 Social Function items. Finally, the NIH PROMIS Physical Function domain was significantly associated with 1 of the 5 items within the EORTC-30 Physical Function subscale (P = .04) (**Table 3**).

In caregivers, similar items were matched across domains and scores compared from NIH PROMIS domains of Sleep Disturbance, Sleep-Related Impairment, Social Activity, Social Role, Depression, and Anxiety with the following CQOLC items: Social Function (4 items), Sleep (1 item), Depression (2 items), and Anxiety (1 item). The authors identified 1 significant correlation between the NIH PROMIS Anxiety domain and 1 subscale item that addressed Anxiety within the CQOLC (P = .04). All other associations between the NIH PROMIS and CQOLC were not found to be significant (**Table 4**).

Exit Survey Results

A pen-and-paper exit survey was used to assess the feasibility of using the iPod Touch, and participants' thoughts and feelings about the individual surveys. One of the 10 patients required a proxy for entering data into the iPod Touch because of fatigue and difficulty visualizing the iPod Touch screen. This patient was read the questions, and data entry was completed by a research assistant. Seventy percent of patients and 100% of caregivers agreed or strongly agreed that they liked taking the surveys on the iPod Touch devices in comparison with a pen-and-paper survey. Four patients and 4 caregivers stated that the iPod Touch was either a little or very difficult to use at first but became easier to use with practice, and 60% of patients and caregivers reported that the iPod Touch was easy or very easy to use. All patients and caregivers reported that they liked the NIH PROMIS survey, although 4 patients and 1 caregiver stated that the number of questions seemed excessive. All patients either agreed or strongly agreed that they liked the EORTC-30, and all caregivers either agreed or strongly agreed that they liked the CQOLC survey. Written comments included suggestions to use an iPod Touch with a larger screen or possibly an iPad in the future, for easier visibility. One patient verbally expressed frustration during the data-collection process and stated that he felt fatigued after completing numerous items on the NIH PROMIS survey.

688

Table 3
Patient correlation summary between the NIH PROMIS survey and the EORTC measure

	NIH PROMIS Domain								
EORTC Variable	Sleep Disturbance	Sleep-Related Impairment	Pain Behavior	Pain Interference	Social Activity	Social Role	Physical Function	P Value	
Insomnia/ Sleep item 1	0.41	0.61	—	—	—	—	—	.23	.06
Insomnia/ Sleep item 2	0.69	0.56	—	—	—	—	—	.03[a]	.10
Physical function item 1	—	—	—	—	—	—	−0.33	.35	
Physical function item 2	—	—	—	—	—	—	−0.66	.04[a]	
Physical function item 3	—	—	—	—	—	—	−0.42	.22	
Physical function item 4	—	—	—	—	—	—	−0.60	.07	
Physical function item 5	—	—	—	—	—	—	−0.14	.69	
Social function item 1	—	—	—	—	−0.49	−0.42	—	.15	.22
Social function item 2	—	—	—	—	−0.37	−0.20	—	.29	.57
Pain item 1	—	—	0.34	0.37	—	—	—	.34	.29
Pain item 2	—	—	0.54	0.61	—	—	—	.10	.06

Items are expressed as Pearson correlations.
[a] $P<.05$.

Table 4
Caregiver correlation summary between the NIH PROMIS survey and the CQOLC scale

	NIH PROMIS Domain						
CQOLC Variable	Sleep Disturbance	Sleep-Related Impairment	Social Activity	Social Role	Depression	Anxiety	P Value
Social function item 1	—	—	−0.02	−0.18	—	—	.94 .62
Social function item 2	—	—	−0.40	−0.20	—	—	.26 .57
Social function item 3	—	—	0.00	−0.16	—	—	1.0 .65
Social function item 4	—	—	0.34	−0.13	—	—	.34 .71
Sleep	0.60	0.43			—	—	.07 .21
Depression item 1	—	—	—	—	−0.47	—	.17
Depression item 2	—	—	—	—	0.50	—	.14
Anxiety	—	—	—	—	—	0.65	.04[a]

Items are expressed as Pearson correlations.
[a] $P<.05$.

DISCUSSION

In this descriptive, pilot study, the authors attempted to validate use of the NIH PROMIS computer-adaptive survey as a quality-of-life instrument in patients with malignant brain tumors and their caregivers. Scores on the NIH PROMIS and EORTC-30 surveys indicated that patients' overall quality of life was slightly below average, and scores on the NIH PROMIS and CQOLC scales suggested that caregivers' overall quality of life was slightly above average. After a comparison of findings, evidence was found to support a significant relationship between the NIH PROMIS Sleep Disturbance domain and an Insomnia/Sleep Function item on the EORTC-30 ($P = .03$). In addition, the NIH PROMIS Physical Function domain was significantly associated with 1 EORTC-30 Physical Function item ($P = .04$). In caregivers, the NIH PROMIS Anxiety domain was significantly associated with 1 item that addressed Anxiety on the CQOLC survey ($P = .04$). These findings provide some support for validation of components of the NIH PROMIS as a quality-of-life instrument for patients with malignant brain tumors and their caregivers.

Most patient/caregiver dyads reported that they enjoyed using the iPod Touch device to complete the quality-of-life surveys, although for some individuals the small screen size made visualization difficult. In addition, one-fourth of the participants (4 patients and 1 caregiver) indicated that the number of items on the NIH PROMIS survey seemed excessive. These individuals recommended that future researchers might consider limiting the number of items necessary for completion of the NIH PROMIS survey.

Strengths and Limitations

Several limitations must be considered when interpreting the results of this study. One limitation is the use of self-reported data that by nature relies on the participants' voluntary disclosure and recall; as such, the results depend on the ability to recall information accurately. Another limitation is the very small sample size, which limits the power of the study. An increase in sample size may have strengthened the results. Correlational findings are considered a limitation because causal inferences cannot be assumed. This community-based convenience sample was composed primarily of white patients with malignant brain tumors and their caregivers. Inferences to other groups should be made with caution. Future researchers are encouraged to examine whether the present findings are applicable to more ethnically diverse samples. A strength of this study is that at the time of data collection, the use of the iPod Touch to complete quality-of-life surveys was fresh and innovative. This approach enabled the authors to assist patients with functional deficits. However, visibility was limited by the small screen size. Future researchers should consider using a smart device with a larger screen size, such as an iPad. Finally, some participants reported that the NIH PROMIS survey contained an excessive number of items. Future researchers may wish to consider limiting the number of survey items participants are expected to complete.

SUMMARY

To the authors' knowledge, this is the first study that has used a sample of patients with malignant brain tumors and their caregivers to validate components of the NIH PROMIS as a quality-of-life instrument. Findings from this study provide support for associations between the NIH PROMIS Sleep Disturbance domain and a Sleep Function item on the EORTC-30, and the NIH PROMIS Physical Function domain and 1 Physical Function item within the EORTC-30. In caregivers, a significant relationship exists between the NIH PROMIS Anxiety domain and Anxiety on the CQOLC survey. In addition, the use of iPod Touch devices by this population to complete quality-of-life surveys is novel. Future research using a larger, more regionally and ethnically diverse sample is recommended.

ACKNOWLEDGMENTS

The authors would like to thank Tina Bambach, MSN, for serving as a research assistant, Dr Olga Herman, PhD, for conducting the statistical analyses, and Dr Andrew Poe, PhD, for designing the iPod Touch quality-of-life app.

REFERENCES

1. Brain tumor statistics. American brain tumor association web site. 2014. Available at: http://www.abta.org/about-us/news/brain-tumor-statistics/. Accessed March 21, 2015.
2. Schmer C, Ward-Smith P, Latham S, et al. When a family member has a malignant brain tumor: the caregiver perspective. J Neurosci Nurs 2008;40(2):78–84.
3. Schubart JR, Kinzie MB, Farace E. Caring for the brain tumor patient: family caregiver burden and unmet needs. Neuro Oncol 2008;10(1):61–72.
4. Kvale EA, Murthy R, Taylor R, et al. Distress and quality life in primary high-grade brain tumor patients. Support Care Cancer 2009;17(7):793–9.
5. Liu R, Page M, Solheim K, et al. Quality of life in adults with brain tumors: current knowledge and future directions. Neuro Oncol 2009;11(3):330–9.
6. Muñoz C, Juarez G, Muñoz L, et al. The quality of life of patients with malignant gliomas and their caregivers. Soc Work Health Care 2008;47(4):455–78.
7. Weitzner MA, Jacobsen PB, Wagner H Jr, et al. The caregiver quality of life index-cancer (CQOLC) scale: development and validation of an instrument to measure quality of life of the family caregiver of patients with cancer. Qual Life Res 1999;8:55–63.
8. Erharter A, Giesinger J, Kemmler G, et al. Implementation of computer-based quality-of-life monitoring in brain tumor outpatients in routine clinical practice. J Pain Symptom Manage 2010;39(2):219–29.
9. PROMIS: dynamic tools to measure health outcomes from the patient perspective. National Institutes of Health Web site. Available at: http://www.nihpromis.org/default.aspx. Accessed March 21, 2015.
10. Aaronson NK, Ahmedzai S, Bergman B, et al. The European Organization for Research and Treatment of Cancer QLQ-C30: a quality-of-life instrument for use in international trials in oncology. J Natl Cancer Inst 1993;85(5):365–76.

Deep Brain Stimulation for Movement Disorders

Maria A. Revell, PhD, MSN, RN, COI

KEYWORDS

- Deep brain stimulation • Parkinson disease • Movement disorders • Essential tremor

KEY POINTS

- Movement disorders, such as Parkinson disease or essential tremor, are frequently caused by neurologic diseases, but can also be the result of injuries, infections, a variety of autoimmune disorders, or side effects of certain medications.
- Deep brain stimulation (DBS) has been identified as a therapy for Parkinson disease and essential tremor.
- DBS is reversible, adjustable with significant advances compared with medications.

INTRODUCTION

Movement disorders arise from a disruption in the interaction between the central nervous system, nerves, and muscles.[1,2] Movement disorders, such as Parkinson disease (PD) or essential tremor, are frequently caused by neurologic diseases, but can also be the result of injuries, infections, a variety of autoimmune disorders, or side effects of certain medications. Although early stages of both PD and essential tremor may not require treatment, both are characterized by involuntary or impaired movements that frequently become debilitating and progressively disabling. These and many other movement disorders can be crippling and cause a significant reduction in quality of life for affected individuals, impairing an individual's ability to speak, control fine motor skills, and maintain balance while walking.[2] When the effects of these disorders begin to interfere with daily life, patients frequently seek out treatment from their care providers.

At present, there is no cure for PD or essential tremor. However, many interventions have been used to manage symptoms. Interventions for motor symptoms of movement disorders over the past several decades have included both surgical and medicinal options.[3] Therapeutic efficacy of these options has often been shown to be limited and complications include speech impairment,[4] recurring tremors, and permanent disability.[5,6]

More recent medicinal interventions for these disorders have varying degrees of effectiveness and, as with many treatments, have a risk of adverse effects. Side

Tennessee State University, 3500 John A. Merritt Boulevard, Box 9590, Nashville, TN 37209, USA
E-mail address: oshum.mr@gmail.com

Nurs Clin N Am 50 (2015) 691–701
http://dx.doi.org/10.1016/j.cnur.2015.07.014
0029-6465/15/$ – see front matter © 2015 Elsevier Inc. All rights reserved.

effects for medicinal intervention may include dizziness, nausea, or confusion, with more serious side effects including severe vomiting, convulsions, or bone marrow issues. In addition, medicinal interventions are many and varied, often requiring significant dosage adjustments before efficacy is achieved, which has led to the use of complementary and alternative management for some disorders, like PD. These therapies, interventions, treatments, and practices include tai chi, acupuncture, art, music, and expressive therapies.[7]

Deep brain stimulation (DBS) is a surgical intervention in which electrodes are implanted in specific areas of the brain to deliver high-frequency electrical stimulation. The area targeted depends on the disorder being treated. DBS has been studied for treatment of motor disorders largely based on the rationale that these disorders stem from dysfunction in the basal ganglia, or motor, circuit of the brain.[8] DBS has been clinically proved to be more effective than medical therapy in providing patients with meaningful motor function and increased quality of life while significantly reducing the potential for experiencing adverse events.[9]

PARKINSON DISEASE
Presentation and Diagnosis

PD is characterized by degeneration of dopamine-producing nerve cells and is slow and expanding in its progression. The neurotransmitter dopamine is essential in stimulating motor neurons, or cells that control motor function. When dopamine production is inhibited as a result of malfunction or death of these dopamine-producing motor neurons, the neurons become unable to control movement.

Symptoms resulting from this deterioration include tremors of the extremities and face, bradykinesia (slow movements), rigidity of limbs and the body trunk, slurred speech, and impairment of balance and coordination (postural instability). These symptoms often worsen with anxiety. It is estimated that symptoms appear when the production of dopamine is inhibited by 60% to 80%.[10]

With an estimated prevalence of more than 4 million people worldwide, PD is one of the most common neurodegenerative diseases, second only to Alzheimer disease.[11] Although not considered a hereditary condition, PD has been found to be familial and have a 2-fold to 3-fold increase in individuals who have first-degree relatives with the disease.[12,13]

Research supports not only genetic but also environmental factors as contributing causes of PD. Identified environmental factors include extended exposure to various toxins, metals, or solvents. Other risk factors include[14]:

- Age more than 60 years
- Male gender
- Traumatic brain injuries resulting in amnesia or loss of consciousness
- Genetic predisposition

Clinical Management

The current standard for clinical management of early-stage PD is oral levodopa treatment,[11] which shows high success rates in patients with PD. However, early initial treatment of levodopa may require high doses in order to overcome peripheral degradation. Although initial improvement is often seen, increasing doses involve complications, which can include long-term extreme dyskinesia. After dosage modifications, which may include the addition of peripheral decarboxylase inhibitors, degradation of medicinal effect can be reduced, which may result in required long-term lower doses with reduced side effects.[15]

Medical management for patients with late-phase Parkinson symptoms becomes more difficult, because the disease becomes increasingly complicated and debilitating. One issue related to levodopa treatment in late-phase PD is fluctuations in efficacy, otherwise termed wearing off or on-off responses. These episodes are characterized by a reduction in motor function being experienced before initiation of the next dose. The duration of dose efficacy may become increasingly shorter, often causing symptoms to reappear suddenly and unpredictably.[15] These episodes can be disorienting and stressful for patients. However, administration of levodopa intravenously has been shown to reduce these fluctuations, resulting in improved outcomes for patients.

Despite many known medicinal complications and difficulty in dosage management, medications continue to be the main treatment of individuals with PD. In addition, despite the best medical management, many patients continue to experience symptom advancement and appearance of new symptoms.[11] When medical management is ineffective, surgical interventions such as DBS must be considered.

ESSENTIAL TREMOR
Presentation and Diagnosis

Essential tremor (ET) is the most commonly diagnosed movement disorder, affecting an estimated 10 million patients nationwide.[16] It is most frequently characterized by the single symptom of uncontrollable shaking of the extremities. The cause of ET remains unknown.[17]

Most commonly, ET is diagnosed based on family history. Diagnosing essential tremor can be difficult, because symptoms can vary significantly and there are no biological markers for ET.

Although some patients diagnosed with essential tremor report difficulties with balance, bradykinesia is not associated with ET. Reported symptoms of ET include:

- Tremors that are intermittent and asymmetric
- Tremors largely affecting the extremities but that also may affect the head, jaw, lips, or face
- Tremors that resolve during relaxation or sleep
- Tremors that vary significantly in amplitude and are worsened by emotion, hunger, temperature extremes, or fatigue[18]

Clinical Management

As with PD, ET is most commonly treated via medical management. Some patients, with only periodic symptoms, may not opt for medication at all. Patients seeking medical management of their symptoms are most likely to be prescribed either primidone, an anticonvulsant, or propranolol, a β-blocker. These medications have been shown to provide significant improvements in motor management in more than half of the patients studied.[19] Although these medications have been shown to be the most effective, up to 50% of patients either cannot tolerate these drugs or do not experience significant benefit from them.[20] In these cases, there are various other drugs that may be considered as alternatives. DBS may be considered if medicinal management is not successful.

DEEP BRAIN STIMULATION

As diagnoses of PD and ET increased throughout history, the drawbacks to conventional medical treatment became apparent. Significant adverse events and lack of efficacy drove investigation into expanding surgical options for these patients.

DBS has been identified as a therapy for PD and ET that has significant advantages compared with medicinal therapies.[8,21,22]

Scientists have been studying electrical stimulation of the brain for treatment of various ailments throughout history. The study of brain stimulation specifically for the treatment of neurophysiologic disorders in the early nineteenth century provided a significant foundation for the understanding and use of this procedure for therapeutic purposes.[23] Deep electrical stimulation of the brain was subsequently introduced to address various motor and behavioral disorders.

DBS, an expanding neurosurgical intervention, was first developed in 1987 in France while treating patients with ET.[24] This procedure involves the implantation of neurostimulation systems into specific areas in the brain (**Fig. 1**). These electrodes are connected to battery-powered pulse generators that require several replacements during an individual's lifetime. Should other hardware components fail, surgical intervention may be necessary to maintain treatment efficacy. DBS has significant advantages compared with pharmacotherapy in that the procedure is not only more effective but patients experience significantly fewer adverse effects.[8] The success of the treatment of ET using DBS prompted investigation into treatment use for PD.

Permanently implanted DBS devices consist of 3 components: leads, implantable pulse generators, and extension cables. There are 2 DBS leads that are inserted into the brain and extend to the skull surface. The 2 generators are typically located in each infraclavicular area. Extension cables connect each lead to an implanted pulse generator (see **Fig. 1**).

DBS technology is based on the rationale that movement motor disorders exist, at least in part, as a result of motor circuit dysfunctions in the brain.[25] As such, electrical stimulation of specific regions of the brain for treatment of specific movement disorders was investigated. Although the exact mechanism of action for DBS therapy is not fully understood, its use has been proved to significantly improve the lives of patients. Since its development, DBS has been granted approval for both PD and ET, in 1997 and 2002 respectively.[8]

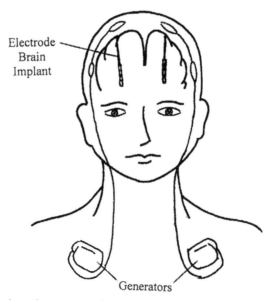

Fig. 1. DBS electrode and generator placement.

Indications and Use

Using high-frequency electrical stimulation to affect neural functions in the brain, DBS has been shown to have long-term efficacy in reducing adverse motor symptoms in patients with both PD and ET.[26] Current protocols for DBS involve implantation of electrodes into strategic points in the brain for treatment of motor dysfunction associated with these disorders. These electrodes are connected to a pulse-generating device similar to a cardiac pacemaker.[8] (see **Fig. 1**).

Indications for DBS currently include medically refractory PD and ET. The area of the brain targeted in therapy varies based on the treated disorder. PD that is tremor dependent is treated with thalamic stimulation (ventralis intermedius), and PD that is dyskinesia predominant is treated with globus pallidus internus stimulation. Other forms of PD that are medically refractory are treated with stimulation of the subthalamic nucleus.

ET is managed with chronic stimulation of the anatomic portion of the brain called the ventralis oralis posterior (Vop; a portion of the thalamus). Some ET is more proximal in origin and may require advancement of electrodes into the zona incerta[27] (**Fig. 2**).

NURSING MANAGEMENT OF PATIENTS WITH DEEP BRAIN STIMULATION

Use of DBS is increasing and it is important that nurses keep abreast of innovative interventions in order to promote the best outcome. As with any surgical procedure,

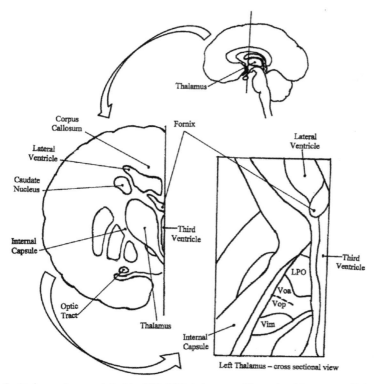

Fig. 2. Brain anatomy related to DBS. LPO, lobus parolfactorius; Vim, ventralis intermedius; Voa, ventralis oralis anterior.

DBS carries with it a potential for transient and permanent complications. Postoperative patient education should include potential complication awareness for patients scheduled to undergo DBS procedures. This information session should be initiated before admission because patients should receive initial postoperative educational information on their decision to have the DBS procedure. It is important to be alert for potential complications after the procedure. Some issues seen in DBS have manifested as movement disorders such as dystonia or dyskinesia. With the number of patients accepting this mode of treatment increasing, nurses must be aware of complications, which include issues related to the surgical procedure, hardware, and stimulation. Early complication intervention is important for the best outcome. It is important that they serve to integrate services between the acute inpatient care and home care.[28]

The nursing protocol for management must include delivery of critical information to move the patient through the decision to self-care (**Fig. 3**). It is imperative that enough educational information is given to patients and families, as appropriate. This information should be in terms that promote understanding and encourage feedback and questioning of the care provider.

Patient Education

Patient preparation begins with education regarding any intervention. This education is required to promote understanding because informed consent is required for surgical interventions. The procedure must be explained to the patient and family if desired, and a signed consent form is mandatory for surgical intervention. It is imperative that all potential complications be explained in order for individuals to make the best informed decisions. Patients must not only be aware of the potential for any complication but also that there is the risk that any experienced complications may be transient or permanent. There are risks for any procedure but the risk/benefit ratio is for the patient to ultimately decide based on information from the health care team. DBS versus best medical care has been studied and results show advantages and disadvantages, as expected[29] (**Box 1**). Several of these adverse events reported in a comparative study had resolved by 6 months.[9]

It is also important to know that risk following DBS can also be associated with preexisting conditions. These conditions include stroke or other neurologic disorders other than ETs and PD, cardiovascular disorders, hepatic failure, renal failure, and diabetes mellitus.[9,30]

Proper patient selection is necessary through retrieval of a thorough history and in-depth physical. A multidisciplinary team evaluation affords identification of the best procedural candidates. Neuroimaging to allow identification of any structural damage and verify placement before surgical intervention,[31] psychological evaluation to validate emotional readiness, self-initiative for compliance adherence and the risk for cognitive decline, and physical therapy to identify physiologic limitations and

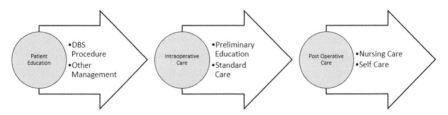

Fig. 3. Protocol for transition from patient education to self-care.

Box 1
Risks and benefits for DBS

Risks

- Headache (<1%)
- Disequilibrium (<1%)
- Death within 1 month of surgical procedure (<1%)
- Stroke (<1%–2%)
- Seizures (<2%)
- Intracranial hemorrhage (3%)
- Infection (3%–5%)
- Hardware malfunction (<5%)

Benefits

- Elimination of efficacy fluctuations
- Potential reduction of pharmacotherapeutic intervention
- Increased efficacy
- Treatment adjustability
- Reversible

---

necessary rehabilitation strategies can improve postprocedural outcomes.[1] Patients should know that this procedure requires adherence to postoperative instructions and follow-up care.

Intraoperative Care

During the DBS procedure, the patient is awake so that motor responses and side effects can be assessed during the procedure.[29] Management of patients psychologically is imperative to avoid anxiety and fear, which may result in movement and actions that could impede the best surgical outcome. As a result, preliminary education must be coupled with standard nursing care to ensure that patients are comfortable throughout the procedure. In addition, nursing care must be provided to ensure that surgical site cleanliness is maintained to avoid infection.

Hemorrhaging

As with most surgeries, bleeding is a potential complication. Although infrequent, bleeding can be potentially serious. This complication may be related to age and can be increased in older patients. In cranial surgery, intracranial hemorrhage is a potential complication and care must be taken to identify this complication early in order to prevent profound debilitation or even death.[32] Symptoms of intracranial hemorrhage include, but are not limited to:

- Change in level of consciousness or alertness (50%)
- Nausea and vomiting (40%–50%)
- Sudden severe headache (40%)
- Seizures (6%–7%)
- Loss of balance or coordinator[33]

Presence of these symptoms should be further evaluated and the physician notified. MRI may be ordered in an effort to obtain proton density images that can give

Table 1 Postoperative care instruction information	
Symptom awareness and management	• There may be some soreness in areas of the head, neck, and chest • There may be swelling around the eyes for a few days following surgery • There may be a microeffect following surgical intervention, which means that symptom severity may increase and decrease sporadically from day to day over several days. This microeffect should self-resolve
Surgical site wound care	• Keep the surgical site clean and dry for at least 5 d • The area around incisions can be gently washed after 5 d • Do not color, perm, or cut hair with clippers for at least 6 wk following surgery • Do not stretch or overextend the neck to prevent pulling of the neck wires • If there is a clear surgical dressing this is removed in 3–5 d by the health care provider • The stitch removal appointment usually includes initiation of the stimulator at that time • Immediate notification is required for a fever >38.6°C (101.5° Fahrenheit) or if redness, swelling, or discharge occurs from the incision site
Medicinal management	• Take all prescribed medications for preexisting health care conditions • Continue to take any blood thinners or aspirin products 2 d after surgery • For mild pain take over-the-counter medications and for more severe pain take prescribed narcotics. Monitor for side effects of narcotics, which can include drowsiness, dizziness, confusion, constipation, nausea, vomiting, difficulty urinating, and itching. If side effects are severe the health care provider should be notified
Physical activities	• The presurgery activity level can be resumed as soon as physically able • Driving can be resumed following verification of driving safety by a friend or family member • Refrain from taking narcotic pain medication while driving
Follow-up care	• Follow-up appointments can occur at 2 wk and 4 wk • Equipment check appointments can occur every 6 to 12 mo • Monitor skin over all hardware sites and report changes such as changes in color, texture, or integrity to the health care provider

a clear picture of bleeding, if present. Although computed tomography or conventional radiology can be used, MRI offers the most sensitive noninvasive mechanism of evaluation for the presence of a bleed and its exact location.

Postoperative Care

Postoperative care begins with a plan to manage the many complications that can occur from DBS. Short-term complications can include weight gain, dyskinesia, speech dysfunction, muscle contractions, visual disturbances, eyelid movement alterations, muscle contractions, and behavioral and cognitive problems. Nursing care should also be given to effectively manage postoperative pain. Long-term complications can include erosion, loss of DBS effect, intermittent stimulation, and tolerance.[34]

Nurses must ensure a thorough understanding of possible complications so that proper assessment for these complications can be performed. It is critical to provide patients and their families with the necessary education regarding the DBS procedure and postoperative care for continued evaluation and management.[29] Patients should understand the short-term and long-term implications of the DBS procedure on their daily lives.

Patient education should cover topics of symptom awareness and management, surgical site wound care, medicinal management, physical activities, and follow-up care (**Table 1**).

SUMMARY

As the age of the population continues to increase, it can be expected that the presentation of patients with movement disorders will continue to grow. Exploring and expanding treatment options for this patient population will be critical in ensuring extended quality of life. DBS offers such benefits. Although this procedure is not a cure for motor diseases, it has been proved to reduce symptom severity and medicinal requirements in patients undergoing the treatment. Unlike ablative therapies, such as thalamotomy and pallidotomy, DBS is reversible and adjustable based on patient symptoms.[1] In addition, the DBS effect has been proved to exist long term with stable stimulation parameters over time.[26] As research on this therapy continues to expand indications for use, it will be critical that health care providers maintain a solid understanding of how to manage these patients.

REFERENCES

1. Machado AG, Deogaonkar M, Cooper S. Deep brain stimulation for movement disorders: patient selection and technical options. Cleve Clin J Med 2012; 79(Suppl 2):S19–24.
2. Wung S. Disorders of function. In: Hannon R, Porth CM, Pooler C, editors. Porth pathophysiology: concepts of altered health States. Philadelphia: Lippincott Williams & Wilkins; 2009. p. 1260–98.
3. Olanow CW, Agid Y, Mizuno Y, et al. Levodopa in the treatment of Parkinson's disease: current controversies. Mov Disord 2004;19:997–1005.
4. Krayenbuhl H, Wyss OA, Yasargil MG. Bilateral thalamotomy and pallidotomy as treatment for bilateral Parkinsonism. J Neurosurg 1961;18:429–44.
5. Nagaseki Y, Shibazaki T, Hirai T, et al. Long-term follow-up results of selective VIM-thalamotomy. J Neurosurg 1986;65:296–302.
6. Jankovic J, Cardoso F, Grossman RG, et al. Outcome after stereotactic thalamotomy for Parkinsonian, essential, and other types of tremor. Neurosurgery 1995;37(4):680–7.
7. Bega D, Zadikoff C. Complementary & alternative management of Parkinson's disease: an evidence-based review of Eastern influenced practices. J Mov Disord 2014;7(2):57–66.
8. Wichmann T, Dostrovsky JO. Pathological basal ganglia activity in movement disorders. Neuroscience 2011;198:232–44.
9. Weaver FM, Follett K, Stern M, et al. Bilateral deep brain stimulation vs best medical therapy for patients with advanced Parkinson disease: a randomized control trial. JAMA 2009;301(1):63.
10. Eller T. Deep brain stimulation for Parkinson's disease, essential tremor, and dystonia. Dis Mon 2011;57(10):638–46.

11. Nolden LF, Tartavoulle T, Porche DJ. Parkinson's disease: assessment, diagnosis, and management. J Nurse Pract 2014;10(7):500–6. Available at: http://www.medscape.com/viewarticle/831281.

12. Gasser T. Genetics of Parkinson's disease. Ann Neurol 1998;44:S53–7.

13. Tanner CM, Ottman R, Goldman SM, et al. Parkinson disease in twins – an etiologic study. JAMA 1999;281:341–6.

14. Tanner CM. Environmental factors and Parkinson's: what have we learned? PDF Newsletter, News and Review 2011. Available at: http://www.pdf.org/environment_parkinsons_tanner. Accessed August 15, 2014.

15. Lundqvist C. Continuous levodopa for advanced Parkinson's disease. Neuropsychiatr Dis Treat 2007;3(3):335–48. Available at: http://www.dovepress.com/articles.php?article_id=912.

16. About essential tremor. International Essential Tremor Foundation. Available at: http://www.essentialtremor.org/about-et/. Accessed February 5, 2015.

17. Hauser RA, McClain TA. Essential tremor. Medscape 2011. Available at: http://emedicine.medscape.com/article/1150290-overview. Accessed February 5, 2015.

18. Burne JA, Hayes MW, Fung VS, et al. The contribution of tremor studies to diagnosis of Parkinson and essential tremor: a statistical evaluation. J Clin Neurosci 2002;9(3):237–42.

19. Primidone and/or propranolol still the drug of choice in treating most patients with disabling essential tremor. Drugs Ther Perspect 2004;20(6):9–13.

20. Nierenberg C. New guidelines for treating essential tremors. American Neurological Association recommends best treatments for the movement disorder. WebMD; 2011. Available at: http://www.webmd.com/brain/news/20111019/new-guidelines-for-treating-essential-tremor. Accessed May 29, 2015.

21. Kalia SK, Sankar T, Lozano AM. Deep brain stimulation for Parkinson's disease and other movement disorders. Curr Opin Neurol 2013;26:374–80.

22. Li Q, Qian ZM, Arbuthnott GW, et al. Cortical effects of deep brain stimulation: implications for pathogenesis and treatment of Parkinson disease. JAMA Neurol 2014;71:100–3.

23. Sironi VA. Origin and evolution of deep brain stimulation. Front Integr Neurosci 2011;5:42.

24. Gardner J. A history of deep brain stimulation: technological innovation and the role of clinical assessment tools. Soc Stud Sci 2013;43(5):707–28.

25. Larson PS. Deep brain stimulation for movement disorders. Neurotherapeutics 2014;11(3):465–74.

26. Rehncrona S, Johnels B, Widner H, et al. Long-term efficacy of thalamic deep brain stimulation for tremor: double-blind assessments. Mov Disord 2003;18: 163–70.

27. Nandi D, Liu X, Bain P, et al. Electrophysiological confirmation of the zona incerta as a target for surgical treatment of disabling involuntary arm movements in multiple sclerosis: use of local field potentials. J Clin Neurosci 2002;9:64–8.

28. Antonini A, Mirò L, Castiglioni C, et al. The rationale for improved integration between home care and neurology hospital services in patients with advanced Parkinson's disease. Neurol Sci 2008;29(Suppl 5):S392–6.

29. American Association of Neuroscience Nurses. Care of the movement disorder patient with deep brain stimulation: AANN clinical practice guideline series. Minneapolis (MN): Medtronic; 2009. Available at: http://www.aann.org/pdf/cpg/aanndeepbrainstimulation.pdf. Accessed April 10, 2015.

30. Medtronic DBS therapy for Parkinson's disease and essential tremor: clinical summary. Minneapolis (MN): Medtronic; 2013. Available at: http://manuals.medtronic.com/wcm/groups/mdtcom_sg/@emanuals/@era/@neuro/documents/documents/contrib_181407.pdf. Accessed May 2, 2015.
31. Benabid AL, Chabardes S, Mitrofanis J, et al. Deep brain stimulation of the subthalamic nucleus for the treatment of Parkinson's disease. Lancet Neurol 2009; 8(1):67–81.
32. Ben-Haim S, Asaad WF, Gale JT, et al. Risk factors for hemorrhage during microelectrode-guided deep brain stimulation and the introduction of an improved electrode design. Neurosurgery 2009;64(4):754–64. Available at: http://www.brown.edu/Research/asaad/neurosurgery2009benhaim.pdf.
33. Liebeskind DS. Intracranial hemorrhage clinical presentation. Medscape 2014. Available at: http://emedicine.medscape.com/article/1163977-clinical. Accessed April 15, 2015.
34. Günther Deuschl G, Herzog J, Galit Kleiner-Fisman G, et al. Deep brain stimulation: postoperative issues. Mov Disord 2006;21(S14):S219–37.

Diabetes Mellitus Standards of Care

Lucy Mays, DNP, APRN, FNP-BC, CNE*

KEYWORDS

- Diabetes mellitus • Glycemic goals • Care of the hospitalized diabetic patient
- Diabetes self-management education

KEY POINTS

- Care of the patient with diabetes can be complex and requires an interdisciplinary approach with an active patient role.
- Roles of the nurse related to the care of patients with diabetes include promoting health, disease prevention, providing patient care, and promoting patient compliance by simplifying self-care.
- Diagnostic criteria and treatment goals for diabetes mellitus are provided.
- Hypoglycemia increases mortality and should optimally be prevented and treated when it occurs.
- Diabetes self-management education is a necessary and reoccurring part of effective management of diabetes.

INTRODUCTION

Diabetes mellitus is a chronic illness that is complex, with multiple contributing factors and complications.[1] There are various types of diabetes mellitus, including but not limited to type 1 diabetes resulting from beta cell destruction that results in a lack of insulin secretion, type 2 diabetes resulting from a progressive defect in insulin secretion in combination with insulin resistance, and gestational diabetes mellitus.[1] Care of the patient with diabetes can be complex and requires an interdisciplinary approach with an active patient role.[1] Guidelines for the management of diabetes are frequently complex and lengthy. Translating evidence-based guidelines into nursing practice is necessary for promotion of positive patient outcomes. Nurses are a critical component in the care of patients with diabetes. Nurses are responsible for monitoring glucose levels, administering hypoglycemic agents,[2] providing patient education,[3] and monitoring for complications.[4] Overall, the roles of the nurse related to the care of patients

Disclosure Statement: The author has nothing to disclose.
St. Claire Regional Primary Care, Morehead State University, CHER 201G, 316 West Second Street, Morehead, KY 40351, USA
* Route 460, Box 57, Denniston, KY 40316.
E-mail address: l.mays@moreheadstate.edu

Nurs Clin N Am 50 (2015) 703–711
http://dx.doi.org/10.1016/j.cnur.2015.08.001
0029-6465/15/$ – see front matter © 2015 Elsevier Inc. All rights reserved.
nursing.theclinics.com

with diabetes include promoting health, disease prevention, providing patient care, and promoting patient compliance by simplifying self-care.[4] Furthermore, because discharge planning for diabetic patients should begin at admission,[1] the nurse should be aware of guidelines related to diabetes care and diabetes self-management.

IMPACT OF DIABETES MELLITUS

The World Health Organization (WHO) estimated that 9% of adults worldwide suffer from diabetes.[5] The incidence of diabetes mellitus is rising in the United States. The number of individuals diagnosed with diabetes rose from 5.6 million in 1980 to 20.9 million in 2011.[6] It is projected that an additional 8.1 million individuals have diabetes but are undiagnosed.[7] The incidence of diabetes in increasing more dramatically for patients with lower educational levels and among the black population.[6]

Diabetes also increases the incidence of morbidity and mortality. There is an increased incidence of hypertension, dyslipidemia, myocardial infarction, stroke, eye disease, kidney disease, and lower limb amputation in patients with diabetes.[6] Diabetes ranks as the seventh leading cause of mortality in the United States.[6]

Diabetes incurs significant financial expenditures. Diabetes was the second leading cause of hospitalization in 2010.[6] In 2012, it was estimated that the cost of diabetes was $245 billion. These expenditures included $176 billion for direct medical care and $69 billion for indirect medical costs (reduced productivity, absenteeism, and early mortality).[8]

DIAGNOSTIC CRITERIA

The American Association of Clinical Endocrinologists and American College of Endocrinology (AACE/ACE)[9] and the American Diabetes Association[1] (ADA) have similar guidelines regarding the diagnostic criteria for diabetes mellitus. ADA guidelines regarding diagnosis of prediabetes (increased risk for diabetes) includes the following criteria.

- A1C 5.7-6.4%
- Fasting plasma glucose 100–125 mg/dL (5.6–6.9 mmol/L)
- 2-h plasma glucose (75 mg oral glucose tolerance test)[1]

ADA guidelines regarding diagnosis of diabetes includes the following criteria.

- A1C $\geq$6.5%
- Fasting plasma glucose $\geq$126 mg/dL (7.0 mmol/L)
- 2-h plasma glucose $\geq$200 mg/dL (11.1 mmol/L)
- Random plasma glucose $\geq$200 mg/dL (11.1 mmol/L)
- Classic hyperglycemic symptoms[1]

Screening for gestational diabetes mellitus (GDM) is recommended, between 24 to 28 weeks of gestation, for pregnant women without diagnosed diabetes.[1] A 75 g oral glucose tolerance test (OGTT) includes measurement of a fasting glucose and glucose measurement at 1- and 2-hour intervals. Diagnosis of GDM includes the following criteria:

- Fasting glucose: $\geq$92 mg/dL
- 1 h OGTT: $\geq$180 mg/dL
- 2 h OGTT: $\geq$ 153 mg/dL[1]

INITIAL EVALUATION

A comprehensive medical evaluation of all patients diagnosed with diabetes should be completed at the initial provider visit.[1] This comprehensive medical evaluation includes a complete medical history, physical exam, laboratory evaluation and re-ferrals to other medical professionals as appropriate.[1]

TREATMENT GOALS

Treatment goal recommendations from the ADA and AACE/ACE are also similar. ADA[1] treatment goals for the general population with diabetes mellitus include the following criteria.

- A1C ≤7% for most; <6.5% for select healthy individuals; <8% for individuals with severe hypoglycemia or certain comorbidities
- Preprandial glucose 80–130 mg/dL (4.4–7.2 mmol/L)
- Peak postprandial glucose <180 mg/dL (<10.0 mmol/L)
- Blood Pressure <140/90 mmHg for most; <130/80 for some healthy individuals[1]

Treatment goals for diabetic patients during pregnancy vary slightly from the general population. ADA glycemic targets patients with GDM include preprandial of no more than 95 mg/dL (5.3 mmol/L) and either 1-hour after meal no more than 140 mg/dL (7.8 mmol/L) or 2-hour after meal no more than 120 mg/dL (6.7 mmol/L)[1]

Women who have diabetes mellitus prior to pregnancy have the following ADA rec-ommendations regarding glycemic goals:

- Premeal, bedtime, and overnight glucose 60 to 69 mg/dL (3.3–5.4 mmol/L)
- Peak postprandial glucose 100 to 129 mg/dL (5.4–7.1 mmol/L)
- A1C <6.0%[1]

PHARMACOLOGIC MANAGEMENT

A complete overview of pharmacologic management for diabetes is beyond the scope of this article. Insulin therapy for patients with type 1 diabetes includes both basal in-sulin (intermediate or long-acting by injection or rapid acting insulin with a pump) and prandial insulin or insulin with meals. This requires several injections daily for adequate glycemic control.[1] Metformin is recommended for patients with type 2 diabetes unless it is not tolerated or contraindicated.[1] Patients with type 2 diabetes frequently require insulin therapy when oral pharmacologic management is not effective.[1] Insulin therapy may also be initiated in the type 2 diabetic if the A1c is greater than 9.0% and the pa-tient has symptoms of hyperglycemia[9] (increased thirst, frequent urination).[10] It is very important to balance carbohydrate intake with prandial insulin in order to achieve adequate glycemic control and to avoid hypoglycemia.[1] The nurse must be aware of insulin onset of action, peak, and duration in order to provide safe and effective in-sulin administration.

Pharmacologic management of diabetes during pregnancy is slightly different than other populations. Insulin is the standard treatment for diabetes during pregnancy. Some oral agents including glyburide and metformin have been used during preg-nancy without negative effects in some patients.[9]

CARE OF THE HOSPITALIZED DIABETIC PATIENT

The ADA and AACE/ACE recommends different glycemic goals for critically ill patients versus healthier patients. Glucose of 140 to 180 mg/dL (7.8–10 mmol/L) is the goal for critically ill patients treated with insulin.[1,9] It is important to prevent hypo-glycemia, because hypoglycemia is associated with higher rates of mortality within the hospitalized patient population.[1,9,11] A lower glucose goal of 110 to 140 mg/dL

(6.1–7.8 mmol/L) can be used for healthier patients if they do not experience hypoglycemia.[1]

MANAGEMENT OF HYPOGLYCEMIA

Hypoglycemia (blood glucose <70 mg/dL or 3.9 mmol/L) can result from an imbalance of nutritional intake, hypoglycemic agents, organ function, release of counter-regulatory hormones, and physical activity.[9] Hypoglycemia has been associated with increased mortality, cardiac arrhythmias, myocardial ischemia, and increased utilization of health care resources.[9] The incidence of hypoglycemia increases with the use of insulin, glinides, and sulfonylureas, or any addition to the existing hypoglycemic medication regimen.[9] Iatrogenic causes of hypoglycemia could include reduced oral intake or nothing by mouth status, lack of synchronization of insulin therapy with meals, intravenous administration of dextrose reduction, decreased/interrupted enteral feedings, and corticosteroid dose reduction.[1] Nurses should be aware of and monitor for symptoms of hypoglycemia, which include but are not limited to tremor, hunger, diaphoresis, paresthesias, cognitive dysfunction, behavioral change, seizure, and coma.[9] Nurses should be particularly vigilant for hypoglycemia in patients who have certain chronic illnesses (renal disease, liver disease, heart failure), infection/sepsis, and malignancy.[1] Identifying causes of hypoglycemia and preventing additional episodes of hypoglycemia[1] are nursing priorities.

Because hypoglycemia can result in coma and death,[1,9] it is extremely important that patients and family members be taught about the signs and symptoms of hypoglycemia. Unfortunately, many patients do not experience symptoms of hypoglycemia and are considered to have hypoglycemia unawareness (HU).[12] Elder patients may have altered symptoms of hypoglycemia,[9] so nurses must be very observant for hypoglycemia in elders with diabetes. Patients who have drastic alterations in glucose levels may also have higher levels of HU.[9] It is imperative that nurses assist in identifying patients with HU and to promote development of awareness of symptoms related to hypoglycemia. Furthermore, family members of patients with HU require information regarding HU, management of hypoglycemia, and emotional support.[13]

Management of hypoglycemia includes 15 to 20 g of oral carbohydrate in patients who are conscious and can tolerate oral intake. The glucose level should be reevaluated in 15 minutes and carbohydrate readministered if hypoglycemia still exists.[1] Glucagon or intravenous dextrose can be administered to patients with hypoglycemia who are unconscious or cannot tolerate oral intake of carbohydrates.[12] Most health care facilities have a hypoglycemia protocol[1] that nurses can follow for patients experiencing hypoglycemia.

DIABETIC KETOACIDOSIS AND HYPEROSMOLAR HYPERGLYCEMIC STATE

Management of patients with diabetic ketoacidosis (DKA) and hyperosmolar hyperglycemic state (HHS) requires provider expertise and vigilant nursing management. The ADA outlines the most recent management of hyperglycemic crisis guidelines in "Hyperglycemic Crises in Adult Patients with Diabetes."[14] Management of DKA and HHS includes but is not limited to managing dehydration and electrolyte imbalance, acidosis and hyperglycemia.[14]

PSYCHOSOCIAL ASPECTS

Emotional health is an integral component of diabetes self-management and care.[1,9] Social/psychosocial issues can negatively impact outcomes in patients with diabetes. Components of social/psychosocial assessment should include but not be limited to the following: affect/mood, expectations for outcomes and medical management, quality of life, and resources (social, emotional, financial). Common disorders to screen for include depression, anxiety, eating disorders, cognitive impairment, and distress related to diabetes.[1] All patients with diabetes should be assessed in an ongoing manner for social/psychosocial issues.[1,9]

NUTRITIONAL GUIDELINES

The ADA[1] emphasizes the need for individualized medical nutrition therapy (MNT) in order to reach individual treatment goals. Furthermore, the ADA[1] recommends that a registered dietitian with expertise in MNT provide patient education. Specific MNT goals for the hospitalized patient include provision of adequate caloric intake to meet metabolic needs, optimal glycemic control, and discharge planning that includes follow-up care.[1] **Table 1** outlines an adaptation of AACE/ACE[9] nutritional recommendations for patients with diabetes.

Table 1
American Association of Critical Care Nurses/American College of Endocrinology healthful eating recommendations for patients with diabetes mellitus

Topic	Recommendation
General eating habits	Eat regular meals and snacks; avoid fasting to lose weight Consume plant-based diet (high in fiber, low calories/glycemic index, and high in phytochemicals/antioxidants) Understand nutrition facts label information Incorporate beliefs and culture into discussions Use mild cooking techniques instead of high-heat cooking Keep physician-patient discussions informal
Carbohydrate	Explain the 3 types of carbohydrates-sugars, starch, and fiber, and the effects of health for each type Specify healthful carbohydrates (fresh fruits and vegetables, legumes, whole grains); target 7–10 servings per day Lower-glycemic index foods may facilitate glycemic control (glycemic index score <55 out of 100: multigrain bread, pumpernickel bread, whole oats, legumes, apple, lentils, chickpeas, mango, yams, brown rice), but there is insufficient evidence to support a formal recommendation to educate patients that sugars have both positive and negative health effects
Fat	Specify healthful fats (low mercury/contaminant-containing nuts, avocado, certain plant oils, fish) Limit saturated fats (butter, fatty red meats, tropical plant oils, fast foods) and trans fat; choose fat-free or low-fat dairy products
Protein	Consume protein in foods with low saturated fats (fish, egg whites, beans); there is no need to avoid animal protein Avoid or limit processed meats
Micronutrients	Routine supplementation is not necessary; a healthful eating meal plan can generally provide sufficient micronutrients Specifically, chromium; vanadium; magnesium; vitamins A, C, and E; and CoQ10 are not recommended for glycemic control Vitamin supplements should be recommended to patients at risk of insufficiency or deficiency

Adapted from American Association of Clinical Endocrinologists and American College of Endocrinology. Clinical practice guidelines for developing a diabetes mellitus comprehensive care plan–2015. Endocr Pract 2015;21(Suppl 1):13. Available at: https://aace.com/files/dm-guidelines-ccp.pdf; with permission.

PHYSICAL ACTIVITY GUIDELINES

Physical activity is beneficial in reducing cardiovascular risk factors, improving physical function, improving feelings of well-being, and reducing fall/fracture risk.[1,15] Physical activity also decreases insulin resistance, decreases glucose levels and helps maintain a healthy weight.[9]

ADA[1] recommendations for physical activity follow:

- Children with diabetes or prediabetes should be encouraged to engage in at least 60 minutes of physical activity each day.
- Adults with diabetes should be advised to perform at least 150 minutes per week of moderate-intensity aerobic physical activity (50%–70% of maximum heart rate), spread over at least 3 days per week with no more than 2 consecutive days without exercise.
- Evidence supports that all individuals, including those with diabetes, should be encouraged to reduce sedentary time, particularly by breaking up extended amounts of time (>90 min) spent sitting.
- In the absence of contraindications, adults with type 2 diabetes should be encouraged to perform resistance training at least twice per week.

The United States Department of Health and Human Services (USHHS) provides age-related guidelines that encourage older adults to "be as physically active as their abilities and conditions allow."[15] The USDHHS also recommends that adults with disabilities "should engage in regular physical activity according to their abilities and should avoid inactivity."[15] Furthermore, persons with disabilities should consult their provider regarding appropriate physical activity for individual conditions.[15]

DIABETES SELF-MANAGEMENT EDUCATION

Diabetes self-management education needs to be individualized, comprehensive, and frequently reinforced. Lifestyle changes necessary to manage diabetes should be personalized to the individual patient's lifestyle, health-related behaviors, and medical conditions.[1,9] Discharge planning prior to hospital discharge of the patient should include the following components as outlined by the ADA:

- Identification of the health care provider who will provide diabetes care after discharge
- Level of understanding related to the diagnosis of diabetes, self-monitoring of blood glucose, and explanation of home blood glucose levels
- Definition, recognition, treatment, and prevention of hyperglycemia and hypoglycemia
- Information on consistent eating patterns
- When and how to take blood glucose-lowering medications, including insulin administration (if going home on insulin)
- Sick day management
- Proper use and disposal of needles and syringes[1]

Management of children and adolescents with diabetes requires involvement of the interdisciplinary health care team, parents, grandparents, and other individuals involved with the child or adolescent such as teachers and coaches. Maintaining frequent communication among all these parties is necessary to promote adequate glucose management. Other developmental concerns should also be addressed depending upon the needs of the individual child or adolescent.[9]

AACE/ACE further recommends that patients with diabetes be taught about avoidance of use of tobacco products.[9] All patients with diabetes should receive a comprehensive program of diabetes self-management education (DSME) at diagnosis, with reinforcement of DSME as appropriate.[1,9] Educating patients regarding foot care (eg, avoiding trauma, washing feet, nail care) has been found to be helpful in preventing diabetic foot ulcers.[16] It is also the role of the nurse to assess for and report any skin changes or decreased foot sensation.[4]

Nurses should also ensure that diabetic patients who are discharged from the hospital have needed equipment, supplies, and prescriptions. The ADA recommends that patients be discharged with the following necessary items:

- Insulin (vials or pens), if needed
- Syringes or pen needles, if needed
- Oral medications, if needed
- Blood glucose meter and strips
- Lancets and lancing devices
- Urine ketone strips (type 1 diabetes)
- Glucagon emergency kit (insulin-treated patients)
- Medical alert application/charms[1]

SICK DAY MANAGEMENT

Individuals with diabetes need to be taught how to manage their diabetes on sick days. Frequent monitoring of blood glucose levels is needed. Patients taking insulin should check their glucose every 2 or 3 hours.[9] Patients should be encouraged to continue taking their medications as a general rule. Basal insulin should still be administered, and short-acting insulin should be administered as appropriate for food intake and glucose level. Carbohydrate-free fluids should be used to maintain hydration. Additional fluid is needed for patients with vomiting and/or diarrhea.[9] Patients with symptoms of DKA should see their health care provider immediately or go to the emergency room. Symptoms of DKA include

- Thirst
- Polyuria
- Glucose greater than 250 mg/dL
- Ketones present in urine
- Fatigue
- Dry skin
- Nausea/vomiting
- Abdominal pain
- Breath with fruity odor
- Confusion[17]

IMMUNIZATIONS

The ADA recommends that both adults and children with diabetes receive standard recommended vaccinations.[1] Further ADA recommendations regarding immunization for patients with diabetes follow:

- Provide routine vaccinations for children and adults with diabetes as for the general population
- Annually provide an influenza vaccine to all patients with diabetes who are at least 6 months of age.

- Administer pneumococcal polysaccharide vaccine 23 (PPSV23) to all patients with diabetes who are at least 2 years of age.
- Adults 65 years of age or older, if previously vaccinated with PPSV23, should receive a follow-up 12 months or later with PCV13.
- Administer hepatitis B vaccination to unvaccinated adults with diabetes who are aged 19 to 59 years.
- Consider administering hepatitis B vaccination to unvaccinated adults with diabetes who are aged 60 years or older.[1]

PREDIABETES MANAGEMENT

Patients with prediabetes should be encouraged to make lifestyle modifications to reduce the chance of developing type 2 diabetes. A healthy diet with caloric reduction when appropriate, in conjunction with regular exercise, should be recommended for patients with prediabetes. Weight reduction activities when appropriate should also be encouraged.[9] Weight loss can be challenging, particularly as lifestyle changes need to be long term. Frequent/regular follow-up is needed to realize significant weight loss.[1]

SUMMARY

Diabetes is a worldwide epidemic that carries a high cost in consumption of health care resources and is associated with increased morbidity and mortality. Nursing care of patients with diabetes is complex and can be challenging. Evidence-based guidelines regarding diabetes management are lengthy and do not always readily translate into hands on nursing care. The nurse must complete a thorough assessment of patients with diabetes, collaborate with the interprofessional team to achieve individual treatment goals, and prevent and effectively manage hypoglycemia. The nurse must begin discharge planning upon admission due to the complex nature of diabetes and the need for patient education and referrals related to diabetes self-management education. Effective management of patients with diabetes requires nurses to be well informed of evidence-based guidelines related to diabetes care.

REFERENCES

1. American Diabetes Association. Standards of medical care in diabetes-2015. Diabetes Care 2015;38(1):S1–93. Available at: http://professional.diabetes.org/admin/UserFiles/0%20-%20Sean/Documents/January%20Supplement%20Combined_Final.pdf.
2. Lange VZ. Successful management of in-hospital hyperglycemia: the pivotal role of nurses in facilitating effective insulin use. Medsurg Nurs 2010;19(1):323–8. Available at: http://eds.b.ebscohost.com/ehost/pdfviewer/pdfviewer?sid=2b0c1ded-adb2-459f-8fe8-d77954b606ea%40sessionmgr110&vid=1&hid=122.
3. Jerreat L. Managing diabetic ketoacidosis. Nurs Stand 2010;24(34):49–56. Available at: http://web.b.ebscohost.com/ehost/pdfviewer/pdfviewer?vid=13&sid=1354631c-1a88-4e73-8866-f95316d5c26b%40sessionmgr113&hid=105.
4. Aalaa M, Malazy OY, Sanjari M, et al. Nurses' role in diabetic foot prevention and care: a review. J Diabetes Metab Disord 2012;11(24):1–6. Available at: http://www.ncbi.nlm.nih.gov/pmc/articles/PMC3598173/pdf/2251-6581-11-24.pdf.

5. World Health Organization. Diabetes. World Health Organization Web site. 2015. Available at: http://www.who.int/mediacentre/factsheets/fs312/en/. Accessed May 26, 2015.
6. Diabetes public health resource. Centers for Disease Control and Prevention Website. 2014. Available at: http://www.cdc.gov/diabetes/statistics/prev/national/figage.htm. Accessed May 19, 2015.
7. Statistics about diabetes. American Diabetes Association Website. 2015. Available at: http://www.diabetes.org/diabetes-basics/statistics/. Accessed May 19, 2015.
8. Economic Costs of Diabetes in the U.S. in 2012. American diabetes Association Website. 2013. Available at: http://professional.diabetes.org/News_Display.aspx?TYP=9&CID=91943&loc=ContentPage-statistics. Accessed May 19, 2015.
9. American Association of Clinical Endocrinologists and American College of Endocrinology. Clinical practice guidelines for developing a diabetes mellitus comprehensive care plan–2015. Endocr Pract 2015;21(Suppl 1):1–86. Available at: https://aace.com/files/dm-guidelines-ccp.pdf.
10. American Diabetes Association. Hyperglycemia (high blood glucose). American Diabetes Association Web site. Copyright 1995-2015. Available at: http://www.diabetes.org/living-with-diabetes/treatment-and-care/blood-glucose-control/hyperglycemia.html. Accessed May 27, 2015.
11. Garg R, Turchin A, Hurwitz S, et al. Hypoglycemia, with or without insulin therapy, is associated with increased mortality among hospitalized patients. Diabetes Care 2013;36:1107–10.
12. McEuen JA, Gardner P, Barnachea DF, et al. An evidence-based protocol for managing hypoglycemia. Am J Nurs 2010;110(7):40–5. Available at: http://ajnonline.com.
13. Lawton J, Rankin D, Elliott J, et al. Experiences, views, and support needs of family members of people with hypoglycemia unawareness: Interview study. Diabetes Care 2014;37:109–15.
14. Kitabchi AE, Umpierrez GE, Miles JM, et al. Hyperglycemic crisis in adult patients with diabetes. Diabetes Care 2009;32(7):1335–43. Available at: http://care.diabetesjournals.org/content/29/12/2739.full.
15. Physical activity guidelines for Americans. U.S. Department of Health and Human Services Web site. 2008. Available at: http://www.health.gov/paguidelines/guidelines/. Updated May 26, 2015. Accessed May 26, 2015.
16. Fujiwara Y, Kishida K, Terao M, et al. Beneficial effects of foot care nursing for people with diabetes mellitus: an uncontrolled before and after intervention study. J Adv Nurs 2011;67(9):1952–62. Available at: http://web.b.ebscohost.com/ehost/pdfviewer/pdfviewer?vid=7&sid=1354631c-1a88-4e73-8866-f95316d5c26b%40sessionmgr113&hid=105.
17. Sick-day rules for managing diabetes. American Diabetes Association Web site. Available at: Copyright 2015. Available at: http://www.diabetesforecast.org/2013/oct/sick-day-rules-for-managing-diabetes.html. Accessed May 20, 2015.

Innovations in Cardiovascular Patient Care: Transcatheter Aortic Valve Replacement

Melanie McGhee, MSN, RN, ACNP-BC

KEYWORDS

- TAVR • SAVR • Aortic valve stenosis • Bicuspid aortic valve • Heart failure

KEY POINTS

- Aortic valve disease is one of the most common and serious valvular disorders and is not reversible through medicinal intervention.
- Aortic valve disease includes bicuspid valve disease and calcific valve disease which progresses on a continuum.
- The option of the transcatheter aortic valve replacement (TAVR/TAVI) offers the high risk surgical patient a treatment for critical aortic stenosis where there used to be none.
- In order for long term success and to lessen complications of the inpatient stay; a multidisciplinary approach that includes nursing is critical.

INTRODUCTION

Heart disease is the leading cause of death in men and women, killing about 610,000 people in the United States annually, which represents 1 in 4 deaths.[1] Although coronary disease is the most common type of heart disease, valvular disease is increasing, especially in individuals more than the age of 65 years because of the predominance of degenerative conditions in this age group. Aortic stenosis (AS) and mitral regurgitation account for 3 in 4 cases of valvular disease, which makes the estimated overall prevalence of valvular disease 2.5%.[2]

Aortic valve disease is one of the most common and most serious of the valvular disorders. No medications can reverse aortic valve disease but medications can be used for symptom management. When medications fail to manage aortic valve disease, other procedural options are explored. These procedural treatment options for aortic valve disease include balloon valvuloplasty, aortic valve replacement, and transcatheter aortic valve replacement (TAVR). The TAVR option has increased in popularity. It is important for nurses to have knowledge of this treatment option in order to ensure the best patient outcomes.

St. Thomas Heart at St. Thomas West, 4230 Harding Road, Suite 410 Nashville, TN 37205, USA
E-mail address: mcghee.melanie@hotmail.com

Nurs Clin N Am 50 (2015) 713–723
http://dx.doi.org/10.1016/j.cnur.2015.07.004
0029-6465/15/$ – see front matter © 2015 Elsevier Inc. All rights reserved.

nursing.theclinics.com

ANATOMIC REVIEW

The aortic valve is one of the four heart valves and sits between the left ventricular outflow tract and the ascending aorta. From the left ventricular outlet to the junction with the ascending aortic portion is called the aortic root.[3] This entire structure is anatomically the aortic valve. The normal aortic valve has 3 leaflets that attach to the ventricular and aortic walls. These half-moon–shaped cusps are semilunar in appearance. In a closed position the valve shows triradiating lines of apposition. This position also exposes small dilatations of the proximal aorta, which are 3 sinuses. Two sinuses are origins for the coronary arteries (the anterior or right coronary artery and the posterior or left coronary artery), and the third is the noncoronary aortic sinus. With the aortic valve in the open position, these sinus openings are protected from the pressure of ventricular ejection by the 3 leaflets. The 3 aortic valve cusps vary in size, with the left and right cusps being more equal in size and the posterior cusp slightly larger in two-thirds of the population.

Outward edges of each cusp attach it to the aortic wall. Attachment occurs at the supraortic ridge, which is composed of a thickened aortic wall structure, called the sinotubular junction, which is the functional level of the aortic valve junction. Small spaces called commissures occur between each cusp. The 3 equally spaced commissures surround the aortic trunk. At the location of the right posterior aspect of the aortic root lie the commissures between the left and posterior cusps. The commissure located at the right anterior aspect of the aortic root is between the right and noncoronary cusp. Physiologically valve structure allows diversion of valve stress to be reflected to the aortic wall.[4]

AORTIC VALVE DISEASE

The aortic valve normally has 3 leaflets or cusps. The valve can have altered functioning through 2 mechanisms: (1) stenosis, and (2) insufficiency. A stenotic valve is narrowed and does not fully open. This condition causes obstruction to the outflow of blood from the left ventricle through the aorta during systole. An insufficient valve leaks blood and allows backflow of blood during diastole. An insufficient valve is the most common alteration of aortic valve functioning. Two common causes of AS in the United States are degenerative calcification and a congenital bicuspid aortic valve. Degenerative calcification of the aortic valve occurs with aging. Calcium and scar tissue buildup from rheumatic valve disease are apparent with increasing age. This buildup is called senile degenerative stenosis.[5] Obstruction to outflow causes left ventricular hypertrophy. This hypertrophy results from increased left ventricular workload. Three classic symptoms of AS are dyspnea, angina, and syncope. In order to prevent sudden death, which has a high probability in untreated AS, surgical intervention is required.

AORTIC STENOSIS

AS is not a disease that occurs in 1 stage. It can be viewed on a progressive continuum. The continuum is initiated by aortic sclerosis and moves to severe AS in approximately 10% of patients.[6] Progression of the disease results in thickening and calcium nodules that further promote stress-related damage between the fibrosa and ventricularis.[7,8] These nodules are located within layers of the leaflet bulge that causes restricted leaflet motion during ventricular systole, which causes obstructed left ventricular systolic outflow (**Fig. 1**).

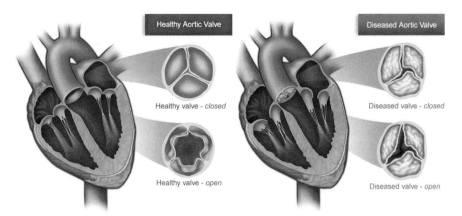

Fig. 1. Normal and diseased aortic valves. (*Courtesy of* Edwards Lifesciences LLC, Irvine, CA; with permission. Edwards and Edwards Lifesciences are trademarks of Edwards Lifesciences Corporation.)

AS is also called calcified aortic valve disease (CAVD). CAVD is an active cellular biological process that can occur with aging. The severity of AS can be graded. This grading system has 3 levels: mild, moderate, and severe. Aortic valve disease is usually found on echocardiogram. The patient is usually sent for an echocardiogram after the appreciation of a murmur on physical examination. The grading of the aortic valve stenosis has specific echocardiographic criteria that include the diameter of the aortic valve, and the peak and mean gradients across the valve via Doppler assessment. Critical aortic valve disease is 100% fatal over time. There are few identified conditions in cardiology that have proved to be as fatal as severe symptomatic AS. Within three years of the onset of angina, syncope, or the symptoms of heart failure, 75% of symptomatic patients are dead unless the outflow obstruction is relieved by aortic valve replacement (AVR) or implantation. Thus, before AVR there is a striking mortality risk of 2% a month. Almost all medical decisions regarding therapy are driven by weighing risks versus benefits of that therapy. Still, many patients with severe AS do not undergo AVR for reasons known and unknown. The risk for AVR regardless of approach is increased in older patients. Advanced age should be viewed as it relates to comorbidities when considering contraindications for AVR. Advanced age alone is not a contraindication for AVR but often physicians, and even patients, are reluctant to have the procedure even with recommendations.[9] Aortic valve replacement is recommended for patients who:

- Need coronary artery bypass grafting surgery, aortic surgery, or other valve surgery concomitantly
- Have an ejection fraction of less than 50% with severe AS
- Are symptomatic with severe AS

Specific echocardiographic criteria inclusive for critical or severe AS include[10]:

- An aortic valve area less than 1.0 cm^2
- A valve area index of less than 0.6 cm^2/m^2
- A mean gradient of greater than 40 mm Hg
- A peak gradient of greater than 64 mm Hg
- A peak velocity greater than 4.0 m/s

It should also be considered that the aortic valve gradients are contingent on the cardiac output, so false-positive or false-negative results could be contingent on whether the heart is in a high-output state (ie, anemia), or a low-output state (ie, heart failure with reduced ejection fraction).

BICUSPID AORTIC VALVE DISEASE

A bicuspid aortic valve (BAV) is a valve that is deformed resulting in only 2 of the 3 functional leaflets. This deformity occurs at birth and has a genetic component.[11] With time and research, it is suggested that BAV disease (BAVD) is caused by a disorder of the connective tissues. It can also cause circulatory system problems, such as problems with the coronary arteries, aortic aneurysms, or aneurysms of the thoracic aorta.

This condition is genetic and can be passed on to first-degree relatives, and typically requires genetic testing of families as a part of a complete treatment. Genetic counseling before pregnancy in these cases is strongly encouraged. AS can eventually result from BAVD. This condition is typically secondary to calcium formation around an already dysfunctional valve. Should this occur, the typical symptoms of AS present, such as chest pain, dizziness, syncope, and/or dyspnea.

CLINICAL FEATURES

AS is usually found in older patients, based on the presentation of a murmur during a normal physical examination. Physiologically, AS is generally asymptomatic until it is moderate to severe. Critical AS is typically characterized by a long period of latency, during which the patient remains largely symptom free. After symptoms develop, functional status rapidly declines as well as life expectancy[12] (see the graph of symptom arrival time and life expectancy) Symptomatic AS has a 50% 2-year survival and a 20% 5-year survival without intervention. Sudden cardiac death can result from critical AS. A combination of both systolic and diastolic heart failure symptoms are an inevitable result of critical AS.

Patients may deny or fail to recognize symptoms by decreasing their levels of exercise to avoid symptoms of angina or dyspnea. This condition is often blamed on the aging process. Angina, syncope, and heart failure are classic symptoms. For these patients, exercise testing may be beneficial to see whether they are truly asymptomatic. Exercise intolerance, ventricular arrhythmias, or hypotension predict an increased mortality and a shorter symptom-free survival. Patients who have been determined to have moderate AS or be truly asymptomatic should be monitored based on progression of symptoms and/or yearly with echocardiogram to evaluate progression of AS. Studies are ongoing to assess whether or not valve implantation for moderate AS should be indicated.[13]

MANAGEMENT OPTIONS FOR AORTIC VALVE DISEASE

After AS is discovered, if the patient is still asymptomatic, the patient can have an excellent survival. However, the risk of sudden cardiac death increases greatly each year. There are also patients recognized to have AS who have heart failure and a depressed ejection fraction. If the increased afterload is from critical AS, the patient should improve dramatically after a surgical or catheter-based intervention, including a substantial increase in ejection fraction after the procedure.

Of the treatment groups of patients with AS, some of the most difficult patients to treat are those with low-flow, low-gradient critical AS. These patients have the poorest prognosis and the highest operative mortality. It is also difficult to make these patients meet the echocardiographic criteria for TAVR/transcatheter aortic valve intervention or implantation (TAVI). Dobutamine stress testing can be helpful here in the absence of coronary disease. These patients sometimes develop a pseudo-AS secondary to the low ejection fraction. The dobutamine assesses the valve using positive inotropic support and increases cardiac output. Contractile reserve in patients with a depressed ejection fraction and the true size of the valve can be evaluated. The presence of a significant contractile reserve is a positive prognostic indicator for patients with possible TAVR/TAVI.

Long-term medical management for AS is not recommended without a prior assessment of the patient's eligibility for any type of valvular intervention, whether it is surgical or catheter based.[14]

WHAT IS A TRANSCATHETER AORTIC VALVE REPLACEMENT?

TAVR is a displacement of the native aortic valve, and the native valve is replaced via a bioprosthetic trileaflet aortic valve percutaneously via balloon catheter. The acronym TAVI can also be used. The most common procedural approach is the transfemoral approach. Other (nontraditional) approaches include transapical, transaxillary, carotid, transaortic (via hemisternotomy), subclavian, and the transcaval approach. The nontraditional approaches are undertaken when the patient has very small femoral arteries or arteries that are unsuitable for a traditional approach.[10]

The first transcatheter aortic valve implantations were performed in animals in 1992. In 2002, Dr Alan Cribier performed the first human TAVR procedure in France.[15] Since this initial procedure a rapid growth has occurred in therapeutics for structural heart disease.[16] The transcatheter approach continues to evolve rapidly as a result of early success and is now indicated as a treatment strategy in both nonsurgical patients and patients who are identified as being in high-surgical-risk groups.[16]

Note that a surgical aortic valve replacement (SAVR) is still the gold standard of treatment and all patients who are determined to be candidates for a TAVR must be declared too high of a surgical risk by 2 cardiothoracic surgeons. For many reasons some patients are declared ineligible for SAVR. For those high-risk surgical patients, the TAVR is a nontraditional but highly effective method of treatment of this life-threatening condition.[11]

TAVR/TAVI is a rapidly evolving field. As of 2013, more than 50,000 implants of TAVR/TAVI valves were done in more than 40 countries.[17] All TAVR procedures are performed in a hybrid operating room suite that is capable of both surgical and catheterization techniques. There are some patients for whom conscious sedation is used. This option is a recent practice and the patients are vigorously vetted to determine their candidacy for conscious sedation. At this time, almost all of these patients still undergo general anesthesia for this procedure.

For a transfemoral TAVR procedure the patient is cannulated similarly to how it would be done during an angioplasty or stent procedure. Occasionally, a femoral cutdown has to be done to use a nondiseased portion of the femoral artery for the procedure. The balloon catheter is then guided into the heart. A compressed transcatheter valve is then loaded onto the balloon and placed directly into the diseased aortic valve. Once in position, depending on the type of valve used, rapid atrioventricular pacing may be performed to decrease the cardiac output. At that time, the valve is deployed via inflation of the balloon. The balloon is then deflated and rapid atrioventricular pacing is terminated. There is a valve that does not require ballooning so, with the use of that particular valve, rapid atrioventricular pacing is unnecessary.

A video of a minimally invasive aortic valve replacement surgery for AS (26:41) can be viewed at http://mdvideocenter.brighamandwomens.org/specialties/cardiovascular/aortic-valve-stenosis-minimally-invasive-aortic-valve-replacement.

The type of transcatheter valve can be facility or physician specific (refer to Figure 5 in Ref.[18]). Each valve has its own learning curve to make it easily deployable for the implanting physician. The type of valve is chosen based on vascular access, the size of the valve that needs to be implanted, the ability to tolerate the rapid atrioventricular pacing, and the ability to tolerate intravenous pyelogram dye, among other reasons. Some patients are able to tolerate the ballooning procedure. Some valves have a higher or lower profile, which may create the necessity of a pacemaker insertion during the hospitalization. Some valves are more prone to paravalvular leak than others and some eventually automatically seal or have a built in cuff or skirt to close to the shape of the native valve, causing less paravalvular leak after the procedure.

Nontraditional approaches to TAVR are done by a cardiothoracic surgeon because these other methods require surgical access. Because TAVR is procedure that is guided by a team approach, an interventional cardiologist is typically on hand for the surgical TAVR procedures and a cardiothoracic surgeon is on hand for the femoral approach procedure.

Patient selection is one of the most important factors to predict good outcomes in TAVR/TAVI. The concept of utility versus futility has been an ongoing debate since Placement of Aortic Transcatheter (PARTNER) valve trial results and the rapid adoption of TAVR worldwide; particularly in Europe.[19,20]

Before the procedure, the patient along with the valve team coordinator must take several steps to ensure candidacy for this procedure. These patients typically have known complications that make them high-risk surgical candidates for SAVR (eg, hemodialysis, neurologic disturbances as a result of cerebrovascular Accident (CVA), atrial fibrillation requiring chronic anticoagulation, previous open chest surgeries). These steps typically include but are not limited to:

- An echocardiogram (which may or may not include a dobutamine stress echo)
- Computed tomography angiography of the chest, abdomen, and pelvis (to verify the size of the annulus of the aortic valve and to determine procedural access)
- Cardiac catheterization (to verify the presence or absence of coronary disease, because this must be addressed before the procedure)
- Pulmonary function testing (to risk stratify and to help determine procedural access)
- Dental examination (to reduce risk of endocarditis)
- Frailty testing (to assess for realistic recovery)
- Society of Thoracic Surgeons (STS) scoring system (to verify open surgical risk)[1]
- Determination to be a high-risk candidate by 2 cardiothoracic surgeons
- Discussion of the case with all available objective data at a multidisciplinary team meeting[10]

After that time, the candidacy for each patient is discussed on a case-by-case basis in a multidisciplinary team meeting. It is similar to a cardiac transplantation team meeting. The goal of the team approach is to use a patient-centered focus to determine and develop the optimal management strategy and plan of care for the patient with severe AS.[11] During the meeting access is determined as well as a plan B for procedure day. It cannot be stressed enough that all patients for

---

[1] The STS scoring system is a tool used to calculate a patient's risk of mortality and morbidities, such as long length of stay, prolonged intubation, and renal failure. The risk calculator incorporates the STS risk models, which are designed to serve as statistical tools to account for the impact of patient risk factors on operative mortality and morbidity.[21]

transcatheter access must be approached in a multidisciplinary fashion. This multi-disciplinary approach helps decrease morbidity, mortality, and (it is hoped) length of stay for the patient.

All high-risk patients come with their own individual set of risks. Some patients are not suitable for TAVR/TAVI. Some patients are temporarily declined and some are permanently declined. In the multidisciplinary team meeting, all patients leave with a plan of care whether it be monitoring with bridge procedures, serial echocardiograms, and follow-up testing or palliation.[12] The transcatheter aortic valve and delivery systems are contraindicated in patients who cannot tolerate an anticoagulation/antiplate-let regimen. The possible contraindications of the valve itself and the delivery system also includes patients who have active bacterial endocarditis or other active infections; known hypersensitivity or contraindication to aspirin, heparin, bivalirudin, ticlo-pidine, clopidogrel, or nitinol (titanium or nickel); sensitivity to contrast media that cannot be adequately premedicated. A preexisting mechanical heart valve in an aortic position can be a contraindication depending on the type of valve in place and the type of valve that is wished to be implanted.[21]

The length of stay is determined based on access, frailty, and level of sedation. A patient with transfemorally accessed TAVR could go home as soon as the next day. The patient leaves the hospital with a 30-day appointment. An echocardiogram is done on the patient at that time to verify valve position and to assess for any para-valvular leak. The patients are assessed for symptoms and frailty tests are usually per-formed again at that time.

RISKS ASSOCIATED WITH TRANSCATHETER AORTIC VALVE REPLACEMENT

All invasive procedures have the possibility of complications. The types of complica-tions specifically associated with TAVR/TAVI can be contingent on how the patient was accessed for the procedure.[22] In general, the risks associated with TAVR are:

- All-cause mortality (3%–5%)
- Stroke or transient ischemic attack (6%–7%)
- Access complications (17%)
- Pacemaker insertion (2%–9% Sapien valve; 19%–43% CoreValve)[2]
- Bleeding
- Prosthetic dysfunction
- Paravalvular leak
- Acute kidney injury
- Other (coronary occlusion, valve embolization, aortic annular rupture)

These risks are all major complications and these are all discussed with patients before the procedure so they may make an informed decision regarding their plan of care. However, it must also always be recognized that patients chosen to un-dergo TAVR/TAVI have been identified as high-risk surgical patients having an STS score of 7% or greater. Ten years ago, withstanding the ballooning of an aortic valve, which was used for palliation, these patients had no other viable op-tions for long term treatment. Some unique patients are identified as bridge to TAVR/TAVI. These patients are symptomatic and frail. They may be offered a balloon valvuloplasty in an effort to ease their symptoms and increase their

---

[2] With greater experience, the overall percentage of permanent pacemaker (PPM) insertion with the CoreValve has decreased with the use of moderate balloon predilatation. It has also been suggested that perioperative conduction abnormalities are transient and do not always require PPM insertion.[23]

Table 1
Complications, cause, care, and considerations for TAVR

Complications	Cause	Care and Considerations
Stroke	Increased age, AV calcification, atherosclerosis of the aorta, balloon valvuloplasty, and THV deployment causing release of microembolic material	Observe patient for neurologic changes. Assess for: • Signs and symptoms of TIA • New-onset AF, which can be associated with late-onset stroke and increased mortality. Continuous telemetry to assess for atrial arrhythmias • Stroke history, because 30-d mortality is 3.5 times higher than for patients without stroke
Cardiac conduction abnormalities	Mechanical disruption of the conduction system by valve deployment	Identify patients who have preexisting conduction abnormalities. • Continue telemetry after procedure until discharge • Administer cautiously atrio-ventricular nodal blocking agents • Resume warfarin or NOAC in addition to ASA 48 h or less after procedure • Resume DAPT early in the setting of recent drug-eluting stent placement
Acute kidney injury	Preexisting renal disease, procedural contrast nephropathy, hypotension, and bleeding	Identify patients at risk early. Even a small increase in the baseline Cr level can be associated with poorer outcomes[26] • Maintain adequate hydration • Consultation of nephrologist early if necessary • Administer renal protective agents such as sodium bicarbonate • Review medication list and discontinue any nephrotoxic agents • During and after TAVR, prevent hypotension • Monitor urine output and creatinine level
Paravalvular leak	THV seating appropriately in the AV annulus, anatomic characteristics and shape of native AV and LVOT	• Assess for signs of hemolysis • Monitor for changes in heart sounds • There is a significant increase in mortality with mild or moderate PVL • Repeat echocardiogram before discharge for compari-son at 30-d follow-up

(continued on next page)

Table 1 *(continued)*		
Complications	**Cause**	**Care and Considerations**
Vascular injury	THV deployment systems with large-caliber sheaths; atherosclerosis of arteries, occult intimal disruptions	Careful blood pressure control (avoiding hypertension and hypotension) • Assess for signs of bleeding, vessel dissection, and tamponade (treat as an emergency) • Assess instrumented limb for vascular insufficiency, groin hematoma, and femoral artery aneurysm
Delirium	Preexisting low-grade delirium, anesthesia, hypotension	• Identify patients at risk early • Use conscious sedation for procedure, if able • Mobilize and resume activity early and limit naps unless already integrated in the patient's daily activities
Prolonged hospital stay	Improper planning, unaggressive management after procedure, unanticipated complications after procedure	• Aggressive postprocedure management to try to facilitate patient's uneventful return to preoperative state • Early inclusion of case management to assess needs after discharge (skilled nursing facility, home health, devices for mobilization) • Early inclusion of physical and occupational therapies to encourage mobilization and assess fall risk

Abbreviations: AF, atrial fibrillation; ASA, acetylsalicylic acid; AV, aortic valve; Cr, creatinine; DAPT, dual anti-platelet therapy; LVOT, left ventricular outflow tract; NOAC, new oral anti-coagulant; PVL, para-valvular leak; THV, transcatheter heart valve; TIA, transient ischemic attack.

Adapted from Ellis MF. Transcatheter aortic valve replacement. Merion Matters, King of Prussia, PA. Available at: http://nursing.advanceweb.com/Continuing-Education/CE-Articles/Transcatheter-Aortic-Valve-Replacement.aspx.

exercise tolerance. After a prescribed time the patient is reassessed and, if the patient has improved in frailty and overall presentation, the patient is again brought to the multidisciplinary meeting to receive TAVR/TAVI. If not, palliation is then offered to the patient.

In patients with the BAV, the TAVR/TAVI is a relative contraindication. It is not widely done in the United States at this time, secondary to BAVs being typically associated with connective tissue disorders and aneurysms. Before the procedure the patient is thoroughly assessed for aneurysms, especially of the ascending aorta. In general, patients should be assessed for ascending, thoracic, and abdominal aneurysms and should generally continue to be assessed on a lifelong basis using computed tomography technology. If the patient is a surgical candidate and has an ascending aneurysm, the patient is typically offered an aortic valve replacement as well as a replacement of the ascending aorta.[24]

POST–TRANSCATHETER AORTIC VALVE REPLACEMENT/INTERVENTION CARE

Postprocedure care of patients having TAVR/TAVI involves close and careful monitoring for postprocedure complications.[25] These complications include but are not limited to stroke, cardiac conduction abnormalities, acute kidney injury, paravalvular leak, valvular injury, delirium, and prolonged hospital stay (**Table 1**).

The outpatient follow-up is scheduled before discharge. An echocardiogram is also done at that time. This ensures a clear plan so the patient is not lost to follow-up. Typically, the patient is seen 30 days after discharge, and then followed again at 6 months and at annual visits after that. The patients are advised that they may need to see their primary care physician or regular cardiologist before their TAVR/TAVI follow-up. This advice is especially common for patients with multiple cardiac comorbidities. A great effort is put into keeping the patient's entire medical team in the loop as to admission, discharge, and disposition.

SUMMARY

With an aging population, valvular disease secondary to degeneration and calcium deposits on the valve will become more common. Critical AS used to be a death sentence for high-risk patients with multiple comorbidities. With the integration of TAVR/TAVI in addition to SAVR, patients are allocated to the intervention that will be the most efficacious and least detrimental to their overall health. While they are inpatients, aggressive and attentive nursing care is crucial to shorten length of stay and decrease possible complications for these patients. A multidisciplinary team approach includes the bedside nurse from the beginning to the end of the patient's hospital course in order to have a successful and less complicated inpatient stay.

REFERENCES

1. Deaths: Final data for 2013. Natl Vital Stat Rep 2015;64(2). Detailed tables released ahead of full report. p. 15. Available at: http://www.cdc.gov/nchs/data/nvsr/nvsr64/nvsr64_02.pdf. Accessed May 1, 2015.
2. Lung B, Vahanian A. Epidemiology of acquired valvular heart disease. Can J Cardiol 2014;30(9):962–70.
3. Piazza N, de Jaegere P, Schultz C, et al. Anatomy of the aortic valvar complex and its implications for transcatheter implantation of the aortic valve. Circ Cardiovasc Interv 2008;1:74–81.
4. Iskandar A, Thompson PD. A meta-analysis of aortic root size in elite athletes. Circulation 2013;127(7):791–8.
5. Nishimura R. Aortic valve disease. Circulation 2002;106:770–2.
6. Cary T, Pearce J. Aortic stenosis: pathophysiology, diagnosis, and medical nonsurgical patients. Crit Care Nurse 2013;33(2):58–72. Available at: http://www.aacn.org/wd/cetests/media/c132.pdf.
7. Saremi F, Achenback S, Arbustini E, et al, editors. Revisiting cardiac anatomy: a computed-tomography-based atlas and reference. Hoboken (NJ): Wiley-Blackwell; 2011.
8. Carabello BA, Paulus WJ. Aortic stenosis. Lancet 2009;373(9667):956–66.
9. Carabello BA. Aortic stenosis: a fatal disease with but a single cure. JACC Cardiovasc Interv 2008;1(2):127–8.
10. Franklin L, Nelson KA, Yuskis D. It's time for a change: transcatheter aortic valve replacement. AAHFN; 2014. p. 1–10.

11. Foffa I, Ait Alì L, Panesi P, et al. Sequencing of NOTCH1, GATA5, TGFBR1 and TGFBR2 genes in familial cases of bicuspid aortic valve. BMC Med Genet 2013;14:44.
12. Minimally invasive aortic valve replacement advantageous for some very elderly patients. The Society of Thoracic Surgeons. Available at: http://www.sts.org/news/minimally-invasive-aortic-valve-replacement-advantageous-some-very-elderly-patients. Accessed May 1, 2015.
13. TCT Daily Staff. Two trials to assess TAVR in moderate risk patients. 2013. Available at: http://www.tctmd.com/show.aspx?id=122078. Accessed May 31, 2015.
14. Bates E. Treatment options in severe aortic stenosis. Circulation 2011;124:355–9.
15. Forrest JK. Transcatheter aortic valve replacement: design, clinical application, and future challenges. Yale J Biol Med 2012;85(2):239–47. Available at: http://www.ncbi.nlm.nih.gov/pmc/articles/PMC3375667/.
16. Smith CR, Leon MB, Mack MJ, et al. Transcatheter versus surgical aortic-valve replacement in high-risk patients. N Engl J Med 2011;364(23):2187–98.
17. Holmes DR Jr, Mack MJ, Kaul S, et al. 2012 ACCF/AATS/SCAI/STS expert consensus document on transcatheter aortic valve replacement: developed in collaboration with the American Heart Association, American Society of Echocardiography, European Association for Cardio-Thoracic Surgery, Heart Failure Society of America, Mended Hearts, Society of Cardiovascular Anesthesiologists, Society of Cardiovascular Computed Tomography, and Society for Cardiovascular Magnetic Resonance. Ann Thorac Surg 2012;93(4):1340–95.
18. Généreux P, Head SJ, Hahn R, et al. Paravalvular leak after transcatheter aortic valve replacement: the New Achilles' heel? A comprehensive review of the literature. J Am Coll Cardiol 2013;61(11):1125–36. Available at: http://content.onlinejacc.org/article.aspx?articleid=1567307.
19. Tang GH, Lansman SL, Cohen M, et al. Transcatheter aortic valve replacement: current developments, ongoing issues, future outlook. Cardiol Rev 2013;21(2):55–76.
20. Reynolds RR, Magnuson EA, Wang L, et al. High-related quality of life after transcatheter or surgical aortic valve replacement in high-risk patients with severe aortic stenosis. J Am Coll Cardiol 2012;60(6):548–58.
21. Short term risk calculator. The Society of Thoracic Surgeons. Available at: http://www.sts.org/quality-research-patient-safety/quality/risk-calculator-and-models. Accessed May 30, 2015.
22. Edwards SAPIEN Transcatheter Heart Valve. Available at: http://www.edwards.com/products/transcathetervalve/Pages/THVcategory.aspx. Accessed May 1, 2015.
23. Thygesen JB, Loh PH, Cholteesupachai J, et al. Reevaluation of the indications for permanent pacemaker implantation after transcatheter aortic calve implantation. J Invasive Cardiol 2014;26(2):98. Available at: http://www.invasivecardiology.com/articles/reevaluation-indications-permanent-pacemaker-implantation-after-transcatheter-aortic-valve.
24. European Society of Cardiology. TAVI feasible in bicuspid aortic valve, study suggests. ScienceDaily 2013. Available at: www.sciencedaily.com/releases/2013/09/130902101900.htm. Accessed May 31, 2015.
25. Elis MF. Transcatheter aortic valve replacement: an evolving option for severe aortic stenosis. Advance Healthcare for Nurses 2015. Available at: http://nursing.advanceweb.com/Continuing-Education/CE-Articles/Transcatheter-Aortic-Valve-Replacement.aspx.
26. Barbash IM, Ben-Dor I, Dvir D, et al. Incidence and predictors of acute kidney injury after transcatheter aortic valve replacement. Am Heart J 2012;163(6):1031–6.

Addressing Tobacco Dependence Through a Nurse-driven Tobacco Intervention Protocol

Tasha Ceass, BA[a],*, Lynn C. Parsons, PhD, MSN, RN, NEA-BC[b]

KEYWORDS

- Health promotion • Smoking • Nursing intervention • Tobacco dependence
- Smoking cessation

KEY POINTS

- Tobacco use is the most prevalent lifestyle behavior that contributes to the largest proportion of preventable disease, disability, and death.
- Mortality among both sexes who smoke in the United States is 3 times higher than among similar people who never smoked.
- Smoking is a primary precursor for cancer, respiratory dysfunction, cardiovascular diseases, and poor fracture healing, because the inhaled components are problematic for several body functions.
- Nurses are in unique positions to converse with patients in an effort to promote smoking cessation interventions.
- Smoking cessation protocols should be initiated that include inpatient and outpatient implementation for best outcomes.
- A nurse-initiated smoking cessation protocol that is collaboratively planned and implemented can reduce morbidity and mortality from smoking-related diseases.

INTRODUCTION

Tobacco use is the most prevalent lifestyle behavior that contributes to the largest proportion of preventable disease, disability, and death. Use of tobacco products is at epidemic proportions in the United States. Estimates retrieved between 2012 and 2013 by the US Centers for Disease Control and Prevention[1] reported that 1 in 5 adults

Disclosure: There are no commercial or financial conflicts of interest and there is no funding source for this article.
[a] Medtronic, Inc., 710 Medtronic Parkway Northeast, Minneapolis, MN 55432, USA;
[b] Department of Nursing, Morehead State University, CHER #201P, 316 West Second Street, Morehead, KY 40351, USA
* Corresponding author.
E-mail address: tashasmithsemail@gmail.com

(50 million) currently used tobacco products every day or some days. Tobacco use was greatest among men, young adults, those living in the Midwest and south, and those with less education.[2] Cigarette smoking resulting in inhalation of tobacco and its by-products is the most common form of tobacco use. Tobacco use results in multiple disease incidences and mortality. Disease incidence includes numerous cancers and chronic diseases (**Fig. 1**).[3]

Mortality among both sexes who smoke in the United States is 3 times higher than among similar people who never smoked. In addition, smoking results in diminished health status, which manifests as an increased risk for adverse surgical outcomes, lost work time (increased absenteeism), and an increase in the use of many medical services.[3] The use of services and cost of health care for smokers is higher and these trends persist into old age.[3] As a profession, nursing has a responsibility to promote care activities that result in health and well-being for all in society. Nurses are the caretakers who are advocates and should promote interventions that include patient education as mechanisms to improve wellness.

Nurses are in unique positions to converse with patients in an effort to promote smoking cessation interventions. They are in contact with patients in acute care facilities, nursing homes, rehabilitation hospitals, clinics, physician offices, and emergency facilities. Being educated about the effects of nicotine and tobacco by-products is imperative. Using this information then allows an effective patient-based intervention program because research has shown an increased probability of stopping smoking for individuals who are offered advice by a nurse.[4]

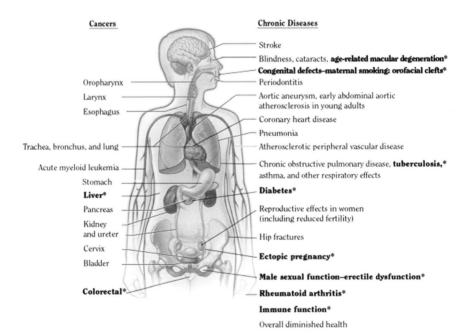

Fig. 1. Health consequences causally linked to smoking. Each condition presented in bold text and followed by an asterisk is a new disease that has been causally linked to smoking in this report. (*From* US Department of Health and Human Services. The health consequences of smoking – 50 years of progress: a report of the Surgeon General. Rockville (MD): Public Health Service; Office of the Surgeon General; 2014. Available at: http://www.surgeongeneral.gov/library/reports/50-years-of-progress/full-report.pdf.)

It is imperative to start from a level of awareness. When caring for individuals who use tobacco products, those individuals must be aware of their potential for withdrawal from nicotine. The use of a collaborative model improves success potential.

PROBLEMS
Smoking and Respiratory Disease

Smoking is a primary precursor for respiratory and cardiovascular diseases because the inhaled components are problematic for several body functions. Cigarette smoke contains a mixture of 4700 chemical compounds, including particulate matter and gaseous components.[5] These compounds cause negative effects at the macrocellular and biochemical levels. Many of these compounds act as oxidants, proinflammatory agents, and carcinogens. They react to cause physiologic changes that result in excessive mucus production as well as bronchial wall chronic inflammatory cell infiltration.[6]

Nicotine is just one of many cigarette chemicals. Nicotine promotes sustained smoking behavior, which increases the desire to smoke and further potentiates the effects of inhaled smoke, tar, carbon monoxide, oxidizing chemicals, and other constituents.[7] It results in thickening of the airway wall. This thickening results from an imbalance of apoptosis and cell proliferation.[8] Active cigarette smoke exposure perpetuates altered physiologic changes and can result in chronic obstructive pulmonary disease (COPD) as well as related diseases that affect the pulmonary tract, such as asthma and allergic rhinitis.[6] COPD is characterized by progressive central airway, peripheral airway, and lung parenchyma inflammation. These inflammatory and structural changes produce remodeling that reduces oxygen availability to body organs and significantly reduces effective functioning. Even after smoking resolution for 1 year airway inflammation does not resolve in individuals with COPD. It is hypothesized that COPD may have an autoimmune component. This response may be an acquired aberrant immune response that results from a defect in the selection, regulation, or death of T or B lymphocytes.[9] This response further perpetuates the physiologic changes that occur in COPD.

Smoking and Cardiovascular Disease

Cardiovascular disease has many risk factors, which include hypertension and family history. Cigarette smoking acts synergistically with these and other risk factors to exponentially increase the risk for cardiovascular morbidity and mortality. Cigarette smoking exposes an individual to nicotine, carbon monoxide, and oxidant gases, which have been identified as causes for cardiovascular disease.[10] Smoking causes sympathomimetic effects, which include increased heart rate and blood pressure. These changes are most prominent shortly after initiating a smoking episode but with continued cigarette use there is a persistent heart rate increase throughout the day.[10]

During a smoking episode, smoke is taken in through mainstream and sidestream mechanisms. Mainstream smoke is taken in through the mouth during active smoking. It consist of 8% tar and 92% other gaseous components. Sidestream smoke is that cigarette smoke emitted from the burning end of the cigarette. This smoke has a higher concentration of toxic gaseous components than mainstream smoke. Both smoke components have effects that are precursors to cardiovascular disease.[11] A significant component of smoke is tar. This element includes polycyclic aromatic hydrocarbons that have been identified to accelerate atherosclerosis.[12]

Smokers have been identified to have changes in platelet functioning and antithrombotic and prothrombotic factors. Research has identified that smoking may decrease availability of platelet-derived nitric oxide and reduce platelet sensitivity to nitric oxide. Nitric oxide is a free radical that has the primary effect of endothelial vasodilation. These changes in nitric oxide lead to increased activation and adhesion.[11,13] Cigarette smokers have higher fibrinogen levels. These levels are directly correlated with the number of cigarettes smoked. Increased blood viscosity and continued inflammatory processes potentiate the prothrombotic process.[11] Cigarette smoking is identified as promoting propagation of thrombus formation as well as reducing the potential for effective dissolution by the body.

Smoking and Cancer

Smoking increases the risk of lung cancer for both men and women by a minimum of 25 times.[1] Inhalation of cigarette smoke contains a mixture of thousands of compounds inclusive of carcinogens. These carcinogens belong to several chemical classes, and include polycyclic aromatic hydrocarbons (PAHs), N-nitrosamines, aromatic amines, aldehydes, volatile organic hydrocarbons, and metals.[14] PAHs are incomplete combustion products and carcinogens that act on a local level in the lungs. N-Nitrosamines are a large carcinogen class and have potent systemic effects. Aromatic amines are combustion products that occur in cigarette smoke. They include the human bladder carcinogens 2-naphthylamine and 4-aminobiphenyl.[14] Aldehydes include formaldehyde and acetaldehyde. Cigarette smoke contains a variety of carcinogens that are capable of causing alterations in tissue integrity.

Enzymes are also involved in activation and detoxification of carcinogens in cigarette smoke. These enzymes include P-450s, glutathione S-transferases (GSTs), UDP-Glucuronosyltransferase (UGT) N-acetyl-transferases, epoxide hydrolases, and sulfotransferases. These enzymes are a few of the wide variety of enzymes that are involved in metabolizing carcinogens found in cigarettes. In addition to these components that affect the onset of lung cancer, genetics and genomics have been instrumental in identifying genome sequencing alterations that result in mutations. These mutations have been found to represent carcinogenic effects associated with tobacco smoking. The most relevant genes in lung cancer include EGFR, KRAS, MET, LKB1, BRAF, PIK3CA, ALK, RET, and ROS1.[15] Missense or nonsense mutations, small insertions or deletions, alternative splicing, and chromosomal fusion rearrangements are some genetic/genomic alterations identified in the literature.[15]

Smoking causes a reduction in respiratory defenses, which include physical barriers, reflex, and the cough response. There are also changes to the epithelial lining of the respiratory tract, alveolar macrophages, and immune responses. These changes alter normal functioning and promote a reduction in protective body responses. Mucus removal is reduced and mucus builds up in airways and lung structures. The resulting impaired mucociliary clearance causes mucus buildup and impaired oxygen transport.[14] These overall macrophysiologic and microphysiologic changes can result in cancers in various respiratory structures.

Other Physiologic Smoking Effects

Fractures can occur from stress or a traumatic incident that causes a break in the bony structure. Fracture healing occurs in stages and restores the bone to its original physical and mechanical properties. Initially under prostaglandin mediation, macrophages, monocytes, lymphocytes, and polymorphonuclear cells infiltrate the bone.[16] Following this, fibrinoblasts begin to lay down stroma that facilitates bone support. Smoking does not promote union for fractures during the healing process.[5] It is recognized as being responsible for nonunion as well as inhibition of fracture healing.[17] Cigarette smoking places the client at risk for osteomyelitis.[18] Tobacco smoke interferes with, and nicotine reduces, functioning of osteoblasts, which inhibits bone repair.

Smoking can be a precursor to pneumonia. Pathophysiologic changes that predispose individuals to cancer also promote susceptibility to bacterial invasion and inflammatory processes that cause pneumonia. Smoking tobacco products weakens the ability for lung components to remove inhaled particles. Smoking also causes irritation of lung tissue through the inhaled toxins and carcinogens, which makes smokers more vulnerable to infection. This irritation is accompanied by mucous gland hypertrophy and immune system damage. As a result of these changes, bacterial infection is more common among smokers and more likely to be a fatal disease in this group of individuals. These changes can be seen in active and passive smokers.[19]

STRATEGIES
Development and Implementation of Smoking Cessation Protocols

Smoking cessation protocols should be initiated that include inpatient and outpatient implementation for best outcomes. Hospitalization offers a unique opportunity for access and implementation of smoking cessation protocols. Clinics, although providing a brief encounter, should be used to gather ongoing information and for continuous assessment of smoking cessation success. All health care contacts should be used to promote smoking cessation and offer continued encouragement and support. Each patient encounter offers an opportunity to potentially improve client health outcomes. Using specific steps to facilitate smoking cessation provides the best potential for success. The following 3 steps individually describe approaches from the nurse and client perspective as well as an important collaborative approach in order to promote success.

- Step 1: nurse focus in planning stages for protocol development. This initial step lays the foundation for subsequent success by the health care team. It begins with recognition of a need for changing client behavior relative to smoking. Identification of a team that is able to collectively correlate areas of expertise allows the development of a protocol that promotes client success. This collaborative committee facilitates development of a foundation for a smoking cessation protocol that is comprehensive. The committee then moves to securing a plan that is time limited but reasonable for the activities required, which include evidence gathering, writing, and implementation (**Fig. 2**).
- Step 2: client focus in planning stages for protocol implementation. Initiation of the client-focused planning stages begins with assessment and awareness. It is important to lay the foundation for smoking cessation inclusive of the desire to stop smoking and identification of perceived barriers. Goals and objectives need to be collaboratively developed and implemented[20] in order for them to be successful because smoking cessation activities require self-governing (**Fig. 3**).
- Step 3: nurse-client merger in implementation of protocol. This step in the protocol process is the most important because it combines the 2 previous steps. Collaborative decisions are the most effective mechanism for protocol success. Initiation of interventions should include a blend of behavioral as well as pharmacologic and/or nonpharmacologic interventions (**Fig. 4**).

Smoking Cessation Strategies

- The Staying Free Program has information available at http://evidencebasedprograms.org/1366-2/staying-free-smoking-cessation-program. This program is a hospital-based intervention program for smokers who desire to

Nurse

- Recognition of the need for a smoking cessation protocol to promote health and wellness.

- Identification of Team Leader for protocol development.
- Selection of Interdisciplinary team.
- Set calendar for timeline from development to initiation.
- Evidence identification for foundation of protocol development.

Initiate Plan for protocol development in setting

- Identify interdisciplinary committee
- Develop step by step plan for process
    - o Investigate and identify current protocols available inside and outside organization related to smoking cessation
    - o Identify desired outcome
    - o Plan for development
        - ▪ develop draft protocol
        - ▪ develop timeline for protocol testing
        - ▪ revise protocol as necessary based on actual performance and collaborative input
        - ▪ determine go-live date for protocol
    - o Plan for acceptance/refusal of various protocol components by client and have alternative options at various steps in the protocol
    - o Develop scripts to promote continuity of approaches by all care providers
    - o Implement based on results of testing phase
    - o Intermittent evaluation of protocol for continued refinement based on research

Fig. 2. Step 1: nurse focus in planning stages for protocol development.

- Assess smoking habits and knowledge level related to harmful effects of smoking
- Assess desire to stop smoking
- Work with client to identify perceived barriers
- Offer options for smoking cessation addressing perceived barriers
- Develop a collaborative plan for smoking cessation that encompasses abilities of client and available resources
  o Educational level of client
  o Individual resources (transportation, etc.)
  o Fiscal resources (insurance vs. self pay for smoking cessation initiatives)
  o Support resources (friends, family members, health care providers, group counseling, coaching activities, telephone counseling)

Fig. 3. Step 2: client focus in planning stages for protocol implementation.

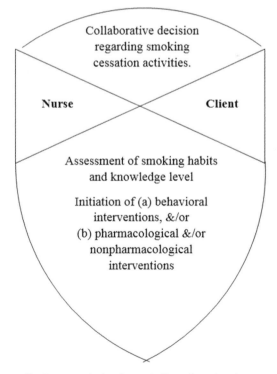

Fig. 4. Step 3: nurse-client merger in implementation of protocol.

initiate smoking cessation while an inpatient. The program incorporates physician information and moves to bedside nurse manager input. Bedside sessions include education, take-home materials, and counseling.[21] Following initial opening sessions there are 4 to 7 telephone nurse counseling sessions of 5 to 10 minutes provided at periodic intervals between 2 and 90 days following hospital discharge. Research has validated this as an appropriate intervention for inpatients who desire to initiate smoking cessation.[22]

- The Treating Tobacco Use and Dependence: 2008 Update, which can be accessed at http://www.ahrq.gov/professionals/clinicians-providers/guidelines-recommendations/tobacco/clinicians/update/treating_tobacco_use08.pdf, is an explicit science-based clinical practice guideline document that validates the importance of smoking cessation along with research-based interventions that may be used. Key recommendations include that health care providers should offer treatments that have been shown to be effective through research, such as individual, group, and telephone counseling. The addition of nicotine-based and non–nicotine-based medications can also promote permanent abstinence. The recommendation of this guide is to use both counseling and medications in an effort to promote success, which has been proved to be more successful than 1 technique alone.[23] This evidence-based document presents meta-analyses that provide validation for recommendations in the guideline.

- Motivational interviewing is a technique that can be used to promote successful smoking cessation.[24–26] Motivational interviewing is an evidence-based approach used to change behavior. It addresses internal ambivalence to change and uses it to promote discovery of people's own interest in making a change in their lives. Ambivalence occurs with many life changes because of conflicting feelings related to the process as well as the outcome. Individuals who are trained to use this ambivalence and guide the client to a positive change can promote positive outcomes for behaviors, such as smoking cessation, that need to be changed in order to promote health and wellness. Motivational interviewing has 4 core principles: (1) express empathy, (2) roll with resistance, (3) develop discrepancy, and (4) support self-efficacy.[27] This type of technique has been proved to promote successful changes in smoking behavior when used by nurses.[24–26]

- Nurse QuitNet, located at https://quitnet.meyouhealth.com/#/, is an evidence-based Internet smoking cessation program for nurses and nursing students. This self-directed online program allows individuals to anonymously use information or self-disclose. The program has been validated to positively affect smoking reduction in nurses. Through research it was identified that nurses who have higher smoking prevalence rates included individual nurses who were less educated and younger nurses (18–24 years old).[28] Web-based programs can be incorporated into smoking cessation protocols and used by organizations to reduce smoking in nurses and nursing students.

SUMMARY/DISCUSSION

Health care professionals are increasingly being held accountable for client outcomes. As medical costs soar it is important that nurses promote healthy lifestyles. It is imperative to facilitate active engagement in behaviors that promote health and prevent illness. Personally tailoring these interventions to client specifics is important.[29,30] The nursing profession should be at the forefront of addressing societal issues that negatively affect health and increase the potential for morbidity and mortality in clients.[31] Smoking is a significant issue that affects not only smokers but persons around them through environmental contamination. Modern health problems are complex and require collective, sustained efforts in order to address them and promote healthy outcomes. Smoking is a changeable health habit that can alter physiologic outcomes for clients and others who interact with them. A nurse-initiated smoking cessation protocol that is collaboratively planned and implemented can reduce morbidity and mortality from smoking-related diseases.

REFERENCES

1. Centers for Disease Control and Prevention. Smoking and tobacco use: Health effects of cigarette smoking. CDC 24/7: saving lives, protecting people. 2014. Available at: http://www.cdc.gov/tobacco/data_statistics/fact_sheets/health_effects/effects_cig_smoking/. Accessed March 15, 2015.
2. Centers for Disease Control and Prevention. Tobacco product use among adults (US). MMWR Morb Mortal Wkly Rep 2014;63(25):542–7. Available at: http://www.cdc.gov/mmwr/preview/mmwrhtml/mm6325a3.htm?s_cid=mm6325a3_w. Accessed March 15, 2015.
3. US Department of Health and Human Services. The health consequences of smoking – 50 years of progress: a report of the surgeon general. Rockville (MD): Public Health Service, Office of the Surgeon General; 2014. Available at: http://www.surgeongeneral.gov/library/reports/50-years-of-progress/full-report.pdf.
4. Rice VH, Stead LF. Nursing interventions for smoking cessation (review). The Cochrane Collaborative. Hoboken (NJ): John Wiley & Sons; 2009.
5. Sloan A, Hussain I, Maqsood M, et al. The effects of smoking on fracture healing. Surgeon 2010;8(2):111–6.
6. Yoshida T, Tudor R. Pathobiology of cigarette smoke induced chronic obstructive pulmonary disease. Physiol Rev 2007;87:1047–82.
7. Smith CJ, Perfetti TA, Garg R, et al. IARC carcinogens reported in cigarette mainstream smoke and their calculated log P values. Food Chem Toxicol 2003;41: 807–17.
8. Colombo G, Clerici M, Giustarini D, et al. Pathophysiology of tobacco smoke exposure: recent insights from comparative and redox proteomics. Mass Spectrom Rev 2014;33(3):183–218.
9. Augusti A, MacNee W, Donaldson K, et al. Hypothesis: does COPD have an autoimmune component. Thorax 2003;58(10):832–4.
10. Benowitz NL. Cigarette smoking and cardiovascular disease: pathophysiology and implications for treatment. Prog Cardiovasc Dis 2003;46(1):91–111.
11. Ambrose JA, Barua RS. The pathophysiology of cigarette smoking and cardiovascular disease: an update. J Am Coll Cardiol 2004;43(10):1731–7.
12. Penn A, Snyder C. Arteriosclerotic plaque development is promoted by polynuclear aromatic hydrocarbons. Carcinogenesis 1988;9:2185–9.
13. Barua RS, Ambrose JA, Srivastava S, et al. Reactive oxygen species are involved in smoking-induced dysfunction of nitric oxide biosynthesis and upregulation of endothelial nitric oxide synthase: an in vitro demonstration in human coronary artery endothelial cells. Circulation 2003;107:2342–7, 40.
14. Centers for Disease Control and Prevention (US); National Center for Chronic Disease Prevention and Health Promotion (US); Office on Smoking and Health (US). How tobacco smoke causes disease: the biology and behavioral basis for smoking-attributable disease: a report of the Surgeon General. Atlanta (GA): Centers for Disease Control and Prevention (US); 2010. 5,

Cancer; Available at: http://www.ncbi.nlm.nih.gov/books/NBK53010/. Accessed March 15, 2015.

15. El-Telbany A, Ma PA. Cancer genes in lung cancer. Genes Cancer 2012;3(7–8): 467–80.

16. Kalfas H. Principles of bone healing. Neurosurg Focus 2001;10(4):E1. Available at: http://www.medscape.com/viewarticle/405699_6.

17. Battersby C, Jermin P, Haigh GA, et al. Clinical experience of smoking cessation advice in hospital trauma units. Eur J Orthop Surg Traumatol 2011;21(10):453–7.

18. Castillo RC, Bosse MJ, Mackenzie E, et al. Impact of smoking on fracture healing and risk of complications in limb-threatening open tibia fractures. J Orthop Trauma 2005;19(3):151–7.

19. Milner D. The physiological effects of smoking on the respiratory system. Nurs Times 2004;100(2):56–9.

20. Cossette S, Frasure-Smith N, Robert M, et al. A pilot randomized trial of a smoking cessation nursing intervention in cardiac patients after hospital discharge. Can J Nurs 2012;22(4):16–26.

21. Hollis J, Lichtenstein E, Vogt T, et al. Nurse-assisted counseling for smokers in primary care. Ann Intern Med 1993;118(7):521–5.

22. Miller N. Translating smoking cessation research findings into clinical practice: the "Staying Free" Program. Nurse Res 2006;55(4S):S38–43.

23. Treating Tobacco Use and Dependence. Agency for Healthcare Research and Quality, Rockville (MD): 2013. Available at: http://www.ahrq.gov/professionals/clinicians-providers/guidelines-recommendations/tobacco/clinicians/update/index.html. Accessed December 12, 2014.

24. Efraimsson EO, Fossum B, Ehrenberg Ö, et al. Use of motivational interviewing in smoking cessation at nurse-led chronic obstructive pulmonary disease clinics. J Adv Nurs 2012;68(4):767–82.

25. Mujika A, Forbes A, Canga N, et al. Motivational interviewing as a smoking cessation strategy with nurses: an exploratory randomised controlled trial. Int J Nurs Stud 2014;51(8):1074–82.

26. Hettema JE, Hendricks PS. Motivational interviewing for smoking cessation: a meta-analytic review. J Consult Clin Psychol 2010;78(6):868–84.

27. Case Western Reserve. Motivational interviewing. Center for Evidence-Based Practices. 2011. Available at: http://www.centerforebp.case.edu/practices/mi. Accessed February 18, 2015.

28. Bialous SA, Sarna L, Wells M, et al. Characteristics of nurses who used the internet-based Nurses QuitNet® for smoking cessation. Public Health Nurs 2009;26(4):329–38.

29. Rowa-Dewar N, Ritchie D. Smoking cessation for older people: neither too little nor too late. Br J Community Nurs 2010;15(12):578–82.

30. Dawal A, Anstey KJ. Interventions for midlife smoking cessation: a literature review. Aust Psychol 2011;2011(46):190–5.

31. Carlebach S, Hamilton S. Understanding the nurse's role in smoking cessation. Br J Nurs 2009;18(11):672–6.

Bedside Reporting
Protocols for Improving Patient Care

Teresa D. Ferguson, DNP, RN, CNE[a],*, Teresa L. Howell, DNP, RN, CNE[b]

KEYWORDS

- Bedside reporting • Hand-off • Shift-to-shift nursing report • Patient-centered care
- Change-of-shift report • Patient safety and bedside reporting
- Patient safety goals and the Joint Commission

KEY POINTS

- Traditional shift reporting involves passing key information about the patient's care to the oncoming shift of nursing personnel.
- The Joint Commission recommendations include a standardized method for "hand-off" communications to engage nursing professionals in sharing significant information and apportioning time to engage in dialogue about the patient.
- Benefits of bedside reporting include patients taking an active role in their care, dynamic dialogue between patients and their care team, increased patient and family satisfaction with care delivery, decreased patient and family apprehension, increased nursing accountability, enhanced teamwork, and decreased potential for errors.
- Address challenges of bedside reporting that include potential violation of the Health Insurance Portability and Accountability Act: compromise of patient privacy and confidentiality, patients in semiprivate rooms or in multiple-bed wards.
- Research supports bedside reporting as a best-practice standard for medical-surgical and rehabilitation units; however, further investigations need to be done, especially in specialty areas such as the emergency department, critical care unit, and labor and delivery/postpartum units.

Bedside reporting at shift change has evolved since the mid-1990s. In the past, shift reporting took place in a conference room with the charge nurse giving the report to the oncoming shift. In addition, the shift report was delivered through audio recording of the patient's pertinent information.[1] These reporting mechanisms did not include face-to-face reporting of patient information, nor did it allow for questions to occur between health professionals. Information contained in this article shares the mechanism

Disclosure Statement: The authors have nothing to disclose.
[a] Department of Nursing, St. Claire Regional Medical Center, 222 Medical Circle Drive, Morehead, KY 40351, USA; [b] Department of Nursing, Morehead State University, 316 West Second Street, CHER 201, Morehead, KY 40351, USA
* Corresponding author.
E-mail address: t.ferguson@moreheadstate.edu

0029-6465/15/$ – see front matter © 2015 Elsevier Inc. All rights reserved.

for "hand-off" bedside reporting protocols, articulates the benefits and challenges with this system, elaborates on supportive research, and shares requirements made by The Joint Commission (TJC) for bedside reporting that include the active involvement of patients in their plan of care.[2]

BACKGROUND

Nurses, as integral members of the health care team, share essential patient information at the change of shift. The procedures for doing this have steadily evolved since the mid-1990s to include "hand-off" reporting between nurses on both shifts that includes the patient at the center of the communications.[3] Over the years the change-of-shift report has taken many forms. Typically in the 1980s a report was given on each patient to every nurse and ancillary personnel on the unit. In the 1990s, on some units personnel were divided by patient load and a report was only given to the team members who were assigned to their allotted patients. Over the next few years, alongside cost-containment efforts, some units had nurses record their shift report, and the oncoming staff listened to the recording. This approach did not give nurses the opportunity to ask questions, verify, or clarify pertinent information. Fast-forward to 2009 when TJC included shift change in the National Patient Safety Goals (NSPGs), requiring that shift reports include current information about changes in patient condition, care, and treatment.[2(p41)] Today many facilities are actively involved in patient-centered care and are moving hand-off to the bedside, where patients and family can actively participate in the plan of care.

THE JOINT COMMISSION MANDATES

TJC developed NPSGs to improve patient safety.[4] Hospitals and other health care facilities must implement measures or protocols to comply with the NPSGs. The NPSGs 2009 required that current pertinent care, treatment, patient condition, and recent changes in information be included in the bedside report.[5] Inclusion of the patient and significant other in bedside reporting is focused on by NPSG-13 for active immersion of the patient in their care regimen.[2(p41)] Health care organizations must include these mandates as outlined by TJC in protocols or procedures developed for bedside reporting.

BEDSIDE REPORTING DEFINED

The Agency for Healthcare Research and Quality defined "hand-off" as "the transformation of information (along with authority and responsibility) during transitions in care across the continuum; to include an opportunity to ask questions, clarify, and confirm" in the 2006 Team Strategies and Tools to Enhance Performance and Patient Safety (TeamSTEPPS).[6] When patient information is handed off from one nurse to another, transferring the care of the patient to the other nurse including responsibility, accountability, and author, it is defined as "report."[7]

CURRENT RESEARCH FINDINGS

Relocation of shift report to the patient's bedside is supported in current research to enhance patient outcomes and satisfaction with care.[8] Chaboyer and colleagues[1(p32)] found that bedside reporting stimulated nurses to recall information about patients that should be shared with the oncoming nurses to ask questions and seek clarity.

Bedside reporting requires less time than traditional shift-to-shift nursing report. In one study the average time in "hand-off" report was 3 minutes.[9] Another finding was that patients took a more active role in the process than they credited themselves. This study was conducted on 8 surgical units. The use of bedside reporting provides a chance for nurses to observe the patient and the environment during report, and leads to a decrease in medication errors and accidents.[10]

Johnson and colleagues[11] identified that a standardized outline of information is needed for nurses to effectively use bedside hand-off reporting. Many issues were identified that contributed to the information nurses had about patients (varying documentation, lack of distinct plans of care, and inconsistent patterns of communication). Research indicates that the incorporation of protocols using the Situation-Background-Assessment-Recommendation (SBAR) reporting system enhances team communication and safety culture.[12,13] **Box 1** displays an adaptation of SBAR for use in bedside reporting.

Involving patients and families in nurse-to-nurse hand-off promotes patient-centered care and the distribution of information at the point of care, but remains an impediment to nurses.[14] Horowitz and colleagues[15] identified the need to use a validated hand-off evaluation tool to measure staff competency, efficacy of hand-off improvements, and endurance of interventions, and to recognize obstacles and gaps in the hand-off process. More research is needed for specialty areas.

BENEFITS OF BEDSIDE REPORTING

Research supports that there are many positives associated with bedside reporting, including increased patient satisfaction with health care delivery and increased job satisfaction among nurses.[8(p282)] Another benefit found by researchers is that bedside reporting increases accountability, safety, and quality.[7(p1)] Rush[2(p43, 44)] stated that one organization showed improved patient satisfaction scores for 3 patient satisfaction measures after implementation of bedside reporting.

In addition, Baker and McGowan[12(p357)] stated that bedside reporting improves patient satisfaction by allowing patients to ask questions or state any concerns during the report process. Bedside reporting also verifies to the patient that the oncoming nurse is aware of all aspects of the patient's condition and important information related to the plan of care or treatment, which may alleviate the patient's anxiety. With bedside reporting patients feel more involved in their care, which increases compliance with their plan of care.[12(p357)]

Another benefit to bedside reporting is promotion of patient safety through communication of pertinent information, and assessment of the patient and the environment. The oncoming nurse gets to spend at least 5 minutes with the patient during the shift-to-shift nursing report, which allows the nurse to briefly assess the patient's condition and any safety issues before going to the next patient.[12(p355)] Nurses are also able to verify the patient's identification and assess that the patient's bed is in a low, locked position and that the call bell is within reach. **Fig. 1** depicts nurses engaged in shift-to-shift bedside reporting.

According to Dearmon and colleagues,[16] transformation of care at the bedside consists of several components, such as use of pain boards, cell phone communication, bedside reporting, and hourly rounding. Transformation of care at the bedside changed traditional ways of thinking and increased advancements in nursing care.[16(p668)] Moreover, bedside reporting allows nurses to spend more time with the patients and improves communication with other nurses.[16(p674)] Tobiano and colleagues[17] found that bedside reporting gave family members the chance to contribute to the care of the patient and increased the accuracy of communication between health care workers.

Box 1
ED bedside shift report using SBAR(T) format

S	Offgoing Nurse—

Manage Up—"I'm going home now. Samantha will be your nurse for the next shift. I've worked with Samantha for 5 years and I can tell you I'm leaving you in good hands. I always hear such nice things about her from her patients."

Oncoming Nurse—

Introduce self using AIDET (Acknowledge, Introduce, Duration, Explanation, Thank You). Update white board

Check armband while asking patient to state his/her name and date of birth

B	Offgoing Nurse—

Involve patient in change-of-shift report—"I'm about to give your report to Samantha. Please listen so at the end you can ask any questions or fill in any additional information that Samantha will need to know to care for you during her shift."

Give a brief update on patient's chief complaint and what treatments/medications have been provided

Update on any pending tests or treatments (ie, laboratory/radiology)

Discuss any special needs (ie, altered mental status, fall risk, isolation precautions)

Oncoming Nurse—

Ask patient if they have any questions

A	Offgoing Nurse—

Give explanation—"We are going to do a quick physical assessment together since we are changing shifts."

Inform the oncoming nurse of what you have assessed and/or noted during your shift

Include any information or tasks that you have completed

Mention what the oncoming nurse will need to complete or follow-up on

Oncoming Nurse—

Review chart and check documentation

Conduct a quick physical assessment and check all intravenous sites/pumps for accuracy

Assess patient's pain using a pain scale

R	Offgoing Nurse—

Review all orders and plan of care with oncoming nurse (tests, treatments, medication therapy, intravenous sites/meds)

Include relevant medications that have been ordered and any ancillary or support services that are working with the patient, such as respiratory therapy, radiology, social services. Ask the patient "Do you have any questions? Is there anything else the nurse needs to know at this time?"

Oncoming Nurse—

Validate orders/plan of care

Ask any questions of offgoing nurse

T	Thank the patient:

Offgoing and Oncoming Nurse—Before leaving the room, ask the patient the following

Is your pain under control?

Do you understand the *plan of care*?

Do you know what you are waiting for and what will happen next?

Do you have any concerns we can address?

Use closing key words:

Offgoing Nurse—"Samantha will take very good care of you. Thank you for allowing me to care for you today."

Oncoming Nurse—"Is there anything you need right now? I'll be back to check on you in about an hour."

Abbreviations: A, assessment; B, background; R, recommendation; S, situation; T, thank you.
From Baker SJ, McGowan R. Bedside shift report improves patient safety and nurse accountability. Journal of Emergency 2010;36(4):356; with permission.

According to the literature, a standardized change-of-shift report improves patient care outcomes.[2(p41),8(p284),18] Evans and colleagues[8(p284)] found that report at the bedside leads to increased direct care time for patients. In one institution, nurses were able to intervene in a timely manner when a patient's status declined during change-of-shift report at the bedside.[2(p43)] The increased time spent with the patient during shift change allows additional assessment of the condition of the patient. However, receiving report outside a patient's room may lead to missing pertinent changes in the patient's condition, resulting in a negative outcome.[2(p43)]

Another benefit associated with bedside reporting is decreased overtime.[16(p668)] Athwal and colleagues[19] found that using bedside reporting led to a reduction in overtime through completion of change-of-shift report in a timely manner. Evans and colleagues[6(p282)] reported that nurses showed increased job satisfaction through being able to leave their shift on time. In addition, nurses had the opportunity to ask

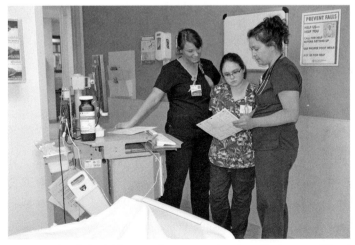

Fig. 1. Nurses engaging in bedside reporting at a regional medical center. (*Courtesy of* Teresa L. Howell, DNP, RN, CNE, Morehead, KY.)

questions during the report process with the previous shift nurse, which also improved their job satisfaction.[6(p282)] A sample survey to measure nurse job satisfaction with bedside reporting on an obstetrics unit is shown in **Box 2**.

CHALLENGES ASSOCIATED WITH IMPLEMENTING BEDSIDE REPORTING

There are several challenges associated with implementation of bedside reporting. Change is difficult for many nurses, which may lead to difficulty in keeping nurses from reverting back to previous methods of shift report.[18]

According to a nurse manager on a women's care unit at a regional medical center, implementation of bedside reporting was initiated approximately 1.5 to 2 years ago on an obstetric/women's care unit without success (L.A. Wallace, RN, MSN, oral communication, 2015). Bedside reporting was unsuccessful at that time because of decreased staff "buy-in" on the unit during the implementation process. This situation

---

Box 2
Sample survey (developed by the authors) for obstetrics unit measuring nurse job satisfaction for hand-off reporting

In an effort to improve shift-to-shift communications between nurses, health team members and patients on the separate units (labor and delivery, nursery, and postpartum), please respond to the following statements. Please circle the answer that best reflects your answer.

1. Sensitive information was shared in the nurse conference room before entering the patient room.

Strongly Agree	Agree	Neutral	Disagree	Strongly Disagree
1	2	3	4	5

2. I had pertinent information to share/give for report.

Strongly Agree	Agree	Neutral	Disagree	Strongly Disagree
1	2	3	4	5

3. The husband/significant other participated in the report.

Strongly Agree	Agree	Neutral	Disagree	Strongly Disagree
1	2	3	4	5

4. The patient was actively involved in the report.

Strongly Agree	Agree	Neutral	Disagree	Strongly Disagree
1	2	3	4	5

5. Communication between shifts is improved with bedside reporting.

Strongly Agree	Agree	Neutral	Disagree	Strongly Disagree
1	2	3	4	5

6. Patient safety has improved with bedside reporting.

Strongly Agree	Agree	Neutral	Disagree	Strongly Disagree
1	2	3	4	5

7. I feel more confident caring for my patient when bedside report is given.

Strongly Agree	Agree	Neutral	Disagree	Strongly Disagree
1	2	3	4	5

8. I receive the information that I need to safely care for my patient during bedside report.

Strongly Agree	Agree	Neutral	Disagree	Strongly Disagree
1	2	3	4	5

9. Bedside reporting improved teamwork on my unit.

Strongly Agree	Agree	Neutral	Disagree	Strongly Disagree
1	2	3	4	5

10. Bedside reporting helped me to identify safety concerns related to my patient.

Strongly Agree	Agree	Neutral	Disagree	Strongly Disagree
1	2	3	4	5

led to nurses reverting to giving their report at the nurses' station (L.A. Wallace, RN, MSN, oral communication, 2015).

In May 2015, L.A. Wallace (oral communication) stated that nurses on the unit were initially resistant to the change in the reporting process. However, recently bedside reporting has been reinstated as the method of providing the shift-to-shift report on the unit. In addition, using bedside reporting cuts out the sharing of personal experiences by nurses during the shift report, decreases the time it takes to report, and improves communication about the patient. At present, the plan is to make a video of nurses on the unit participating in bedside reporting as a training tool for new nurses and as an incentive to make bedside reporting more personable for the nursing staff, which will improve "buy-in" of the nurses on the unit (L.A. Wallace, RN, MSN, oral communication, 2015).

Nurses on the women's care unit use two standardized documents during hand-off communication for labor and delivery and couplet care of the mother/baby. **Figs. 2** and **3** are examples of these documents. One of the labor and delivery nurses stated that a full report is given about the patient at the bedside excluding social services issues (A. Johnson, RN, BSN, oral communication, 2015).

Nurses are able to do a mini-assessment of the patient during report by checking the patient identification bracelet, intravenous site, need for pain medication, dressing changes, and any safety issues. In May 2015, A. Johnson (oral communication) stated that reporting at the bedside made patients feel more included in their plan of care. One barrier noted was that at times it is difficult for patients to participate and focus when multiple family members are in the room during the report.

One of the postpartum nurses stated that bedside reporting eliminates inconsistencies in care from one nurse to another by validating information with night- and day-shift nurses and the patient (C. O'Cull, LPN, oral communication, 2015). As a result of bedside reporting, nurses will be more conscientious about how they leave the patient at the end of the shift. Tasks will be less likely to be left undone because the next shift nurse will be visually aware of the patient's condition and documentation of care from the previous shift.[12(p355)]

Caruso[18(p21)] found that nurses were not comfortable in including patients in the report process. Therefore, it is important to explain the bedside reporting process to patients and the importance of their providing input during the report process.[9(p21)] Patients should be asked if they have any information to share or have any questions regarding their care.[9(p547)] Patient-centered care allows the patient to feel engaged in the change-of-shift report. Timonen and Sihvonen[9(p542)] found that patients had a difficult time understanding the medical terms nurses used during the report process. To eliminate confusion, nurses should report in a manner such that the patient understands what is being discussed.

Providing patient privacy and confidentiality was another challenge associated with bedside reporting. Chaboyer and colleagues[1(p31)] reported that confidential information was discussed away from the patient's room to prevent other people from hearing the conversation during the report process. **Fig. 4** illustrates nurses engaged in sharing sensitive information away from the bedside.

ESTABLISHING A PROTOCOL FOR HAND-OFF BEDSIDE REPORTING

A review of the literature revealed established protocols for hand-off bedside reporting for general medical-surgical and rehabilitation units. However, protocols are needed for specialty areas such as labor and delivery/postpartum, emergency department (ED), and critical care units.

Diagnosis	Allergies	Cervical Exam	BOW	LBM/Foley	IVF/Site	VS/I&O	Diet	
								418

OB History: EDD: _____ G____ ,P____ ,T____ ,Pt____ ,Ab____ ,L_____   Pain Management: _____

Blood Type____ , HIV_____ , Hep B_____ , GBS_____   Rubella:_____   Room after Delivery: _____

Pediatrician:_____ ,   Breast/Bottle   Labs: _____

KC Care: Yes/No

Nursing Communication:_____

Diagnosis	Allergies	Cervical Exam	BOW	LBM/Foley	IVF/Site	VS/I&O	Diet	Room
								419

OB History: EDD: _____ G____ ,P____ ,T____ ,Pt____ ,Ab____ ,L_____   Pain Management: _____

Blood Type____ , HIV_____ , Hep B_____ , GBS_____   Rubella:_____   Room after Delivery: _____

Pediatrician:_____ ,   Breast/Bottle   Labs: _____

KC Care: Yes/No

Nursing Communication:_____

Fig. 2. Sample hand-off report sheet for Labor and Delivery from a regional medical center. (*Data from* S. Sadler, RN, APRN, email communication, 2015.)

Room # _____ Couplet Report Sheet Allergies: _____

Delivery Method Date & Time	Diet	Foley/ I&O	VS	IVF	Activity	Perineal Repair	Sitz Bath/Ice	T-Dap	Birth Certificate	Paternity	Portrait of a promise	D/C Teaching

OB History: EDD: _____ G _____, P _____, T _____, Pt _____, Ab _____, L _____

Blood Type _____, Rhogam Given: _____ HIV _____, Hep B _____, GBS _____

Rubella: _____ Pediatrician: _____

Delivery Complications: _____

Nursing Communication: _____

Diet	VS	HBV	ALGO	Photo	Heart Screen	BP	Newborn Screen	Circumcision	Bili	Cord Clamp	D/C Teaching

Voiding: _____ Stooling: _____ Emesis: _____

Feeding: _____ Nipple Type: _____

Apgar: 1 _____, 5 _____, 10 _____

Neonatal Resuscitative Measures: _____

Nursing Communication: _____

Weight: Birth _____ Day 2 _____ D/C Weight _____

Fig. 3. Sample hand-off form for Labor and Delivery from a regional medical center. (*Data from* S. Sadler, RN, APRN, email communication, 2015.)

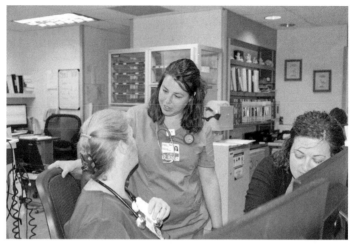

Fig. 4. Nurses sharing sensitive patient information away from the bedside at a regional medical center. (*Courtesy of* Teresa L. Howell, DNP, RN, CNE, Morehead, KY.)

There are several important factors to consider during the implementation of bedside reporting, the first of which is to formulate a committee including nurses and other team members to be involved in the development and implementation of bedside reporting on the unit.[20] This committee will be involved with the development of new policies or updating current policies or protocols related to the implementation process, training of staff, and evaluating the nurses after implementation of bedside reporting. Second, the committee must develop specific goals that are measurable. Third, a clear plan must be developed indicating how bedside reporting should occur on the unit. Fourth, a tool must be developed for use during the shift-to-shift report which is specific to the patient population on the unit. The last step is to educate the nurses and implement the bedside reporting process on the unit.[20(p10)]

Establishing a protocol for nurses to follow during the transition to bedside reporting using patient-centered care is necessary to make nurses more comfortable with the process, in addition to ascertaining that all pertinent information is being shared during the hand-off. In 2008, Chaboyer and colleagues[21] reported using a 5-step process to implement bedside reporting: preparation, introduction, information exchange, patient involvement, and safety scan. A sample protocol for hand-off bedside reporting on an obstetrics unit is provided in **Box 3**.

During the preparation phase, it is important to notify the patient 20 minutes before the report will occur. During this time, the nurse can obtain consent from the patient, allowing any family or visitors into the room during the report. Facilities must protect patient information as outlined by the Health Insurance Portability and Accountability Act.[22] Confidentiality may be compromised when patients are in semiprivate rooms, or by having other persons in the room for hand-off bedside reporting. The facility can have the patient sign a release allowing the husband or significant other to remain in the room during the report to protect the facility from a liability standpoint. Nurses may discuss sensitive information at the nurses' station before entering the patient's room.[18(p21)] In addition, the nurse should assess the patient's pain status and administer medications as needed for patient comfort while the report is taking place. If the patient is comfortable, it will be easier for her to focus on the information and clarify any misconceptions, or ask questions about their care.

Box 3
Sample protocol for hand-off bedside report on an obstetrics unit

Preparation:

1. Nurses are given a team of patients to care for during their shift including labor and delivery, postpartum, and newborns

2. An electronic reporting tool is given to each nurse, which gives a brief overview of all the patients on the obstetric unit

3. Patients are informed within a specific time-frame that the bedside report will take place in about 20 minutes

4. Obtain consent for family or visitors to remain in the room during the bedside report from the patient. Nurses will ask family or visitors to step out of the room as needed

5. Assess pain level and administer pain medications as needed

Introduction:

1. The nurse from the outgoing shift introduces the oncoming nurse to the patient and family

2. Other team members may be present, such as nursing assistants

Information Exchange:

1. Use SBAR (Situation, Background, Assessment, and Recommendation) as a reporting tool

2. Use terms and language that the patient and family will understand. Avoid medical terms

Patient Involvement:

1. Give the patient and family the opportunity to ask questions related to care, clarify information exchanged, or give other important information

2. Confidentiality must be maintained by discussing confidential information at the nurses' station outside of the patient room

Safety Scan:

1. The nurses review the patient, environment, and electronic patient record

2. Patient: Assess any incisions or dressings, drains, catheters, intravenous lines

3. Environment: Assess intravenous pumps or other pumps, oxygen, suction equipment, call bell in reach, bed in low and locked position

4. Electronic Health Record: Review Medication Administration Record to verify all medications have been given and documented correctly; vital signs, intake and output, and so forth is documented; risk assessments for skin breakdown and falls are completed

5. Allow the oncoming nurse to verify information and ask questions

6. Update white boards if applicable

7. Notify patient when the bedside report is complete

Adapted from Chaboyer W, McMurray A, Wallis M. Standard operating protocol for implementing bedside handover in nursing. Queensland (Australia): Griffith University; 2008; with permission.

The introduction involves the current shift nurse introducing the oncoming nurse and providing a brief statement about the nurse to help establish rapport between the patient and the nurse assuming care. The two nurses verify the identification of the mother and baby via the mother/baby identification bracelets.

During the information exchange, the report consists of using SBAR and giving a brief history of the labor and delivery, including complications such as hemorrhage, laboratory data, and any other significant information. If the mother has an intravenous site, it should be checked for patency and signs of infiltration or infection, and the type and rate of intravenous infusion noted. Nurses should verify that allergy and medication information is current. It is vital to assess any incisions, drains, tubes, or catheters that may be present. A brief assessment and report for the newborn should consist of respiratory distress, color, temperature, circumcision site (if applicable), and cord site in addition to feeding and elimination pattern. It is important to discuss pain and pain management, and any teaching that has been completed or is necessary.

During the patient involvement stage, the patient is encouraged to clarify information or ask questions about themselves or the newborn. The final stage is the safety scan. The nurse assesses safety measures, including having the bed in a low, locked position, the call bell within reach, and the safety bracelet intact for allergies and/or risk of a fall if applicable. In addition, the nurse observes any pumps, oxygen, or suction equipment being used.

SUMMARY

TJC has mandated NPSGs to facilitate treatment of patients' current conditions and promote communication between health professionals and hospitalized patients. Validation of accurate information between shifts promotes patient safety. Another benefit of bedside reporting is the nurses' ability to streamline their work and avoid unnecessary overtime.

Bedside reporting is a pragmatic communication tool to facilitate a current account of the patient's condition. Inclusion of the patient as an integral member of the health team is paramount to promoting health and recovery from illness. Nurses have become more comfortable with the hand-off process with increased use of the system and establishment of hand-off protocols. Health care organizations adopting these protocols report that restructuring end-of-shift reporting has simplified the communication process while simultaneously upholding patient safety standards.

REFERENCES

1. Chaboyer W, McMurray A, Wallis M. Bedside nursing handover: a case study. Int J Nurs Pract 2010;16:27–34.
2. Rush S. Bedside reporting: dynamic dialogue. Nurs Manage 2012;43:41–4.
3. Friesen MA, White SV, Byers JF. Handoffs: implications for nurses. In: Hughes RG, editor. Patient safety and quality: an evidence-based handbook for nurses. Rockville (MD): Agency for Healthcare Research and Quality (US); 2008. Chapter 34. Available at: http://www.ncbi.nlm.nih.gov/books/NBK2649/.
4. Facts about the National Patient Safety Goals. The Joint Commission Website. 2015. Available at: http://www.jointcommission.org/standards_information/npsgs.aspxPublished. Accessed May 28, 2015.
5. Revere A, Eldridge N. JCAHO National Patient Safety Goals for 2007. Topics in Patient Safety. 2007; 7(1). Available at: http://www.patientsafety.va.gov/docs/TIPS/TIPS_JanFeb08.pdf#page=1. Accessed May 29, 2015.
6. King B, Battles J, Baker D, et al. TeamSTEPPSTM: Team strategies and tools to enhance performance and patient safety. ARHQ.gov. 2015. Available at: http://www.ahrq.gov/professionals/quality-patient-safety/patient-safety-resources/resources/advances-in-patient-safety-2/vol3/Advances-King_1.pdf. Accessed May 19, 2015.
7. Alexander A, Fletcher M, Navarro R, et al. Bedside report: Is it the best practice for our patients? ADVANCE for Nurses Website. 2013. Updated April 22, 2013.

Available at: http://nursing.advanceweb.com/Features/Articles/Bedside-Report. aspx. Accessed May 19, 2015.

8. Evans D, Grunawalt J, McClish D, et al. Bedside shift-to-shift nursing report: implementation and outcomes [serial online]. Medsurg Nurs 2012;21(5):281–92.

9. Timonen L, Sihvonen M. Patient participation in bedside reporting on surgical wards [serial online]. J Clin Nurs 2000;9(4):542–8.

10. Griffin T. Bringing change-of-shift report to the bedside: a patient- and family-centered approach [serial online]. J Perinat Neonatal Nurs 2010;24(4):348–55.

11. Johnson C, Carta T, Throndson K. Communicate with me: information exchanges between nurses [serial online]. Can Nurse 2015;111(2):24–7.

12. Baker SJ, McGowan R. Bedside shift report improves patient safety and nurse accountability. Journal of Emergency Nursing 2010;36(4):355–8.

13. Velji K, Baker R, Fancott C, et al. Effectiveness of an adapted SBAR communication tool for a rehabilitation setting. Healthc Q 2008;11(Sp):72–9.

14. Johnson M, Cowin LS. Nurses discuss bedside handover and using written handover sheets. J Nurs Manag 2013;21:121–9.

15. Horwitz L, Dombroski J, Murphy T, et al. Validation of a handoff assessment tool: the handoff CEX [series online]. J Clin Nurs 2013;22(9/10):1477–86.

16. Dearmon V, Roussel L, Buckner EB, et al. Transforming care at the bedside (TCAB): enhancing direct care and value-added care. J Nurs Manag 2013;21: 668–78.

17. Tobiano G, Chaboyer W, McMurray A. Family members' perceptions of the nursing bedside handover [series online]. J Clin Nurs 2013;22(1/2):192–200.

18. Caruso E. The evolution of nurse-to-nurse bedside report on a medical-surgical cardiology unit [serial online]. Medsurg Nurs 2007;16(1):17–22.

19. Athwal P, Fields W, Wagnell E. Standardization of change-of-shift report. J Nurs Care Qual 2009;24(2):143–7.

20. Nurse bedside shift report: implementation handbook. Agency for Healthcare Research and Quality Website. Available at: http://www.ahrq.gov/professionals/systems/hospital/engagingfamilies/strategy3/strat3_implement_hndbook_508.pdf Accessed May 28, 2015.

21. Chaboyer W, McMurray A, Wallis M, et al. Standard operating protocol for implementing bedside handover in nursing. Queensland (Australia): Griffith University; 2008. Available at: http://www.safetyandquality.gov.au/implementation-toolkit-resource-portal/resources/additional-clinical-handover-resources/national-clinical-handover-initiative-tools/griffith-university/Bedside-Handover%20SOP.pdf. Accessed May 29, 2015.

22. Summary of the HIPAA Privacy Rule. U.S. Department of Health & Human Services Web site. 2003. Available at: http://www.hhs.gov/ocr/privacy/hipaa/understanding/summary/privacysummary.pdfLast. Accessed May 29, 2015.

Management of Travel-Related Illness Acquired in Haiti

Michele Walters, DNP, APRN, FNP-BC, CNE

KEYWORDS

- Haiti • Topical diseases • Dengue • Chikungunya • Malaria • Travelers' diarrhea

KEY POINTS

- Management of travel-related diseases acquired in Haiti begins with the identification of tropical diseases that are prevalent in the region.
- Knowledge of various tropical disease incubation periods and presenting symptoms is crucial to ensure rapid triage and management of care.

After the 2010 earthquake in Haiti, many relief aid workers and missionaries traveled to Haiti to offer medical assistance and humanitarian relief efforts. Many of these individuals became ill themselves during their stay in Haiti or upon return home. Approximately 8% of travelers visiting developing countries will seek health care while abroad or after returning home.[1] Many travelers will return home with a fever and associated symptoms. Illness acquired while traveling may be minor and self-limiting or may progress to a life-threatening illness. Health care providers need to take a systematic approach to evaluate individuals traveling to developing regions. Travelers returning from Haiti should be evaluated for several febrile illnesses that are prevalent in the Caribbean. Practitioners should consider differential diagnoses that include dengue, chikungunya, malaria, and travelers' diarrhea.

DENGUE

Dengue is the most prevalent mosquito-borne viral disease throughout the world. The dengue virus is estimated to contribute to 390 million infections each year.[2] Dengue is a febrile illness that is caused by 4 different serotypes of the flavivirus (DENV-1, DENV-2, DENV-3, and DENV-4).[3] All 4 serotypes circulate throughout the Caribbean, with

Disclosure Statement: The author has nothing to disclose.
Center for Health Education and Research, Morehead State University, 316 West Second Street, CHER 201F, Morehead, KY 40351, USA
E-mail address: ma.walters@moreheadstate.edu

Nurs Clin N Am 50 (2015) 749–760
http://dx.doi.org/10.1016/j.cnur.2015.07.013
0029-6465/15/$ – see front matter © 2015 Elsevier Inc. All rights reserved.

DENV-1 and DENV–2 being predominant.[4] The disease is spread by the day-biting *Aedes* mosquitoes.[5] The incubation period may range from 3 to 14 days after exposure to infected *Aedes* mosquitoes. The symptoms with initial infection can be self-limiting to asymptomatic. Sequential infections with the different subtypes will lead to increasing severity in symptoms.

Classic dengue symptoms will present with an acute febrile illness with accompanied symptoms of headache, orbital eye pain, myalgia, arthralgia, nausea, vomiting, diarrhea, lymphadenopathy, and rash.[5] The typical dengue fever can last up to 7 days. The rash is generally noted during the initial infection 2 to 5 days after the onset of fever. A sequential infection with a different subtype generally does not produce the rash. Individuals residing in the endemic region or engaging in extended travel in the endemic region are at higher risk for sequential infections. Sequential infections pose a greater risk of developing severe symptoms of dengue hemorrhagic fever or dengue shock syndrome. The World Health Organization (WHO) suggests the following clinical approach to a dengue classification and levels of severity (**Table 1**).

Rapid diagnostic laboratory testing with combined NS1 antigen and immunoglobulin M (IgM) enzyme immunoassay would be optimal diagnostic tools if available.[6,7] The US Food and Drug Administration (FDA) has approved the IgM enzyme-linked immunosorbent assay (ELISA) for use in the United States. Unfortunately, individuals residing in Haiti typically do not have the option of laboratory testing. Another noninvasive diagnostic test is the tourniquet test. The tourniquet test is a marker of capillary fragility and can be used as a triage tool to differentiate patients suspected of having dengue infection.[8]

How to do a Tourniquet Test

A tourniquet test has the following steps[8]

1. Take the patient's blood pressure and record it (eg, 100/70).
2. Inflate the cuff to a point midway between systolic blood pressure and diastolic blood pressure and maintain for 5 minutes (eg, [100 + 70] ÷ 2 = 85 mm Hg).

Table 1
World Health Organization clinical approach to dengue classification and levels of severity

Probable Dengue	Dengue Warning Signs Leading to Severe Disease	Severe Dengue
Live in/travel to dengue endemic area	Laboratory confirmed dengue with signs of:	Severe plasma leakage leading to:
Fever and 2 of the following criteria:	• Abdominal pain or tenderness	• Shock
• Nausea, vomiting	• Persistent vomiting	• Fluid accumulation with respiratory distress (pleural effusion)
• Rash	• Clinical fluid accumulation	• Severe bleeding
• Aches and pains	• Mucosal bleeding	• Severe organ involvement
• Tourniquet test positive	• Lethargy, restlessness	• Liver: aspartate aminotransferase or alanine aminotransferese ≥1000
• Leukopenia	• Liver enlargement >2 cm	• Central nervous system: impaired consciousness
	• Laboratory: increase in hematocrit concurrent with rapid decrease in platelet count	

From World Health Organization and the Special Programme for Research and Training in Tropical Diseases. Dengue guidelines for diagnosis, treatment, prevention and control. Geneva (Switzerland): World Health Organization; 2009; with permission.

3. Reduce and wait 2 minutes.
4. Count petechiae below antecubital fossa.

A positive tourniquet test is 10 or more petechiae per 1 square inch (**Fig. 1**). If the test is negative and reveals no bleeding, the tourniquet test should be repeated.[8] There are no guidelines as to the frequency of repeated tourniquet testing to identify the presence of dengue.

There are no definitive treatments for the dengue serotypes, and supportive care should be provided for presenting symptoms. Early diagnosis and supportive care preventing dehydration, reducing fever, and monitoring for hemorrhage and vascular permeability have shown to reduce mortality.[9] A preventative approach should be taken to ward off infestation. No vaccines are currently available, although several vaccines are in development, with a chimeric tetravalent vaccine in phase 3 clinical trials.[10] Mosquito control remains the most effective approach for prevention of dengue.

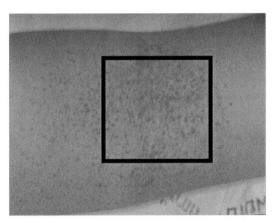

Fig. 1. Positive tourniquet test.

CHIKUNGUNYA

Chikungunya fever (ChikV) is arthropod-borne virus that has previously been endemic to West Africa until 2013, when the virus emerged in the Caribbean islands.[11] ChikV is transmitted via bites from the *Aedes aegypti* or *A albopitus*. The *A aegypti* and *A albopitus* mosquitoes are easily identified due to the white markings found on the legs and body (**Fig. 2**). Both mosquito types can be found throughout the United States, which raises a concern for the transmission of ChikV. In 2014, local transmission of ChikV infection was reported in Florida.[11] Up to this point, the ChikV cases in the United States were in travelers returning from infected regions, which makes it crucial for health care professionals to identify the signs and symptoms of ChikV.

ChikV incubation period can range from 1 to 14 days.[12] ChikV symptoms typically appear between 3 to 7 days, with the onset of a fever that may range from a low-grade temperature to temperatures greater than 101°F. Associated symptoms are fatigue, headache, eye pain, nausea, vomiting, muscle pain, joint pain, and rash. Skin manifestations have been reported in up to 75% of patients.[13] Individuals residing in Haiti presented with a rash within 24 hours after onset of fever. The maculopapular rash had a neuropathic quality that individuals described as a burning or stinging, puretic rash (**Fig. 3**). The rash often involved the palms of the hands and soles of the feet. Marked joint pain in the wrists and hands presented with individuals holding

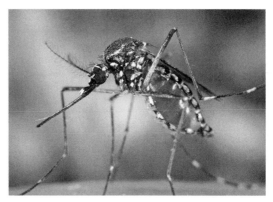

Fig. 2. *A aegypti* mosquito. (*Courtesy of* CDC/ Prof. Frank Hadley Collins, Dir., Cntr. for Global Health and Infectious Diseases, Univ. of Notre Dame.)

them in a flexed position. In addition to the upper extremity arthralgias, the ankles were affected, contributing to a limping gait upon presentation.

There are no vaccines to prevent the spread of ChikV or specific treatment. Care should be taken to rule out dengue infection, as ChikV and dengue have similar clinical presentations. Symptomatic care is the only method of treatment for ChikV. The fever and arthralgias should be treated with acetaminophen until dengue is ruled out to prevent the potential for hemorrhage. Serology is the primary tool for diagnosis by monitoring IgM and IgG antibodies.[13] IgM antibodies will appear within 1 to 12 days and persist up to 3 months. IgG antibodies present 2 weeks following onset of symptoms and may persist for years. In the absence of laboratory, testing the tourniquet test should be utilized to differentiate dengue from ChikV. Once ChikV is identified, nonsteroidal anti-inflammatory drugs appear to offer greater relief from the arthralgia pain. Individuals with chronic symptoms complain of joint polyarthralgias with associated localized edema in the majority of these individuals.[14]

As with dengue, prevention of exposure to infected mosquitoes remains the key. Individuals who return to the United States having traveled to an area with ChikV or develop ChikV symptoms should remain inside during daytime hours for 14 days to prevent infection of the local mosquito population. Notification of local health

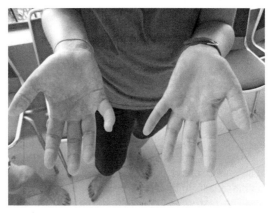

Fig. 3. Chikungunya rash.

departments is requested to assist in tracking infections within the United States and monitor for transmission of the disease. The local health departments report to the US Centers for Disease Control and Prevention (CDC) to maintain geographic distribution reporting of ChikV.[11]

MALARIA

Malaria is a tropical disease that is caused by the *Plasmodium* parasite that infects the female *Anopheles* mosquito.[15] There are 4 kinds of *Plasmodium* malaria parasites that infect humans: *Plasmodium falciparum, P vivax, P ovale*, and *P malariae. P falciparum* is the most serious and may progress rapidly to life-threatening illness within hours of onset of symptoms. Over 1500 cases of malaria are reported to the CDC each year. During 2012, more than half of the reported cases were caused by *P falciparum*.[16] The incubation period of *P falciparum* is 12 to 14 days, with most infections becoming clinically apparent within 1 month after exposure.[17]

Clinical presentation is nonspecific, with a febrile illness with associated symptoms of chills, fatigue, tachycardia, tachypnea, cough, diaphoresis, headache, nausea, vomiting, diarrhea, arthralgias, and myalgias.[15] A physical finding that would separate malaria from other tropical diseases would be the presence of splenomegaly. Microscopic examination of blood smears is commonly used in practice of remote areas as well as in the United States to confirm the malaria diagnosis. Treatment should be guided by 3 main factors of identifying the *Plasmodium* species, the clinical status of the client, and drug susceptibility as determined by geographic area of the infecting species.

Malaria may be classified as uncomplicated or complicated. Uncomplicated malaria can occur with any *Plasmodium* species. *P falciparum* malaria has the greatest potential for severe complications, which include: altered consciousness with or without seizures, severe anemia, hypoglycemia, acute respiratory distress syndrome, shock, metabolic acidosis, disseminated intravascular coagulation, renal failure, and hepatic failure.[18]

The CDC published clinical guidelines that provide treatment tables that can be utilized to guide malaria care.[15] Haiti is in a region where malaria remains susceptible to chloroquine phosphate. Chloroquine phosphate is approved for use in pediatric clients and pregnant individuals. **Table 2** outlines uncomplicated malaria treatment and chloroquine phosphate dosing. Treatment guidelines for complicated malaria and treatment for other regions are available through the CDC. Complicated malaria should be treated with parenteral antimalarial therapy.

Individuals traveling to Haiti should take a chemoprophylaxis agent. Antimalarial therapy should start prior to travel, continue during travel exposure, and follow departure for the recommend treatment time. Chloroquine phosphate may be used for prophylaxis for individuals traveling to Haiti. Chlororquine phosphate is preferred by most traveling to Haiti due to the cost and weekly dosing. Chloroquine should be started 1 to 2 weeks prior to travel.[19] Other antimalarial drugs are available for prophylaxis and recommended for use in chloroquine-resistant areas (**Table 3**).[19]

In addition to malaria chemoprophylaxis, individuals need to take general protective measures to protect against mosquito exposure in affected regions. Minimizing the amount of exposed skin by wearing long sleeves and pants to cover the legs is suggested. The CDC recommends application of products to exposed areas that contain at least 20% DEET.[20] The use of insect repellent (permethrin) on clothing is recommended in high-exposure areas. Insect repellent may be found with camping equipment in most retail stores.

Table 2
US Centers for Disease Control and Prevention uncomplicated malaria treatment guidelines for Haiti

Species	Region	Recommended Adult Dose	Recommended Pediatric Dose (Pediatric Dose Should not be Greater than Recommend Adult Dose)
Uncomplicated malaria/P falciparum or species not identified	Chloroquine-sensitive (Central America west of Panama Canal; Haiti; the Dominican Republic; and most of the Middle East)	Chloroquine phosphate (Aralen and generics)[8] 600 mg base (equal to 1000 mg salt) by mouth immediately, followed by 300 mg base (equal to 500 mg salt) by mouth at 6, 24, and 48 h Total dose: 1500 mg base (equal to 2500 mg salt) OR Hydroxychloroquine (Plaquenil and generics) 620 mg base (equal to 800 mg salt) by mouth immediately, followed by 310 mg base (equal to 400 mg salt) by mouth at 6, 24, and 48 h Total dose: 1550 mg base (equal to 2000 mg salt)	Chloroquine phosphate (Aralen and generics) 10 mg base/kg by mouth immediately, followed by 5 mg base/kg by mouth at 6, 24, and 48 h Total dose: 25 mg base/kg OR Hydroxychloroquine (Plaquenil and generics) 10 mg base/kg by mouth immediately, followed by 5 mg base/kg by mouth at 6, 24, and 48 h Total dose: 25 mg base/kg

Data from Malaria. Centers for Disease Control and Prevention Web site. 2015. Available at: http://www.cdc.gov/malaria/index.html. Accessed May 20, 2015.

Table 3
Drugs used in the prophylaxis of malaria

Drug	Usage	Adult Dose	Pediatric Dose	Comments
Atovaquone-proguanil	Prophylaxis in all areas	Adult tablets contain 250 mg atovaquone and 100 mg proguanil hydrochloride 1 adult tablet orally, daily	Pediatric tablets contain 62.5 mg atovaquone and 25 mg proguanil hydrochloride 5–8 kg: ½ pediatric tablet daily >8–10 kg: ¾ pediatric tablet daily. >10–20 kg: 1 pediatric tablet daily >20–30 kg: 2 pediatric tablets daily >30–40 kg: 3 pediatric tablets daily >40 kg: 1 adult tablet daily	Begin 1–2 d before travel to malarious areas Take daily at the same time each day while in the malarious area and for 7 d after leaving such areas. Contraindicated in people with severe renal impairment (creatinine clearance <30 mL/min). Atovaquone-proguanil should be taken with food or a milky drink Not recommended for prophylaxis for children weighing <5 kg, pregnant women, and women breastfeeding infants weighing <5 kg. Partial tablet doses may need to be prepared by a pharmacist and dispensed in individual capsules, as described in the text
Chloroquine phosphate	Prophylaxis only in areas with chloroquine-sensitive malaria	300 mg base (500 mg salt) orally, once/wk	5 mg/kg base (8.3 mg/kg salt) orally, once/wk, up to maximum adult dose of 300 mg base	Begin 1–2 wk before travel to malarious areas. Take weekly on the same day of the week while in the malarious area and for 4 wk after leaving such areas. May exacerbate psoriasis
Hydroxychloroquine sulfate	An alternative to chloroquine for prophylaxis only in areas with chloroquine-sensitive malaria	310 mg base (400 mg salt) orally, once/wk	5 mg/kg base (6.5 mg/kg salt) orally, once/week, up to maximum adult dose of 310 mg base	Begin 1–2 wk before travel to malarious areas. Take weekly on the same day of the week while in the malarious area and for 4 wk after leaving such areas

(continued on next page)

Table 3
(continued)

Drug	Usage	Adult Dose	Pediatric Dose	Comments
Doxycycline	Prophylaxis in all areas	100 mg orally, daily	≥8 y of age: 2.2 mg/kg up to adult dose of 100 mg/d	Begin 1–2 d before travel to malarious areas Take daily at the same time each day while in the malarious area and for 4 wk after leaving such areas. Contraindicated in children <8 y of age and pregnant women
Mefloquine	Prophylaxis in areas with mefloquine-sensitive malaria	228 mg base (250 mg salt) orally, once/week	≤9 kg: 4.6 mg/kg base (5 mg/kg salt) orally, once/wk >9–19 kg: 1/4 tablet once/wk >19–30 kg: 1/2 tablet once/wk >30–45 kg: 3/4 tablet once/wk >45 kg: 1 tablet once/wk	Begin ≥2 wk before travel to malarious areas Take weekly on the same day of the week while in the malarious area and for 4 wk after leaving such areas. Contraindicated in people allergic to mefloquine or related compounds (quinine, quinidine) and in people with active depression, a recent history of depression, generalized anxiety disorder, psychosis, schizophrenia, other major psychiatric disorders, or seizures Use with caution in persons with psychiatric disturbances or a previous history of depression Not recommended for persons with cardiac conduction abnormalities

From Yellow Book. Center for disease control and prevention. Available at: http://wwwnc.cdc.gov/travel/yellowbook/2014/chapter-3-infectious-diseases-related-to-travel/malaria. Accessed May 20, 2015; with permission.

Table 4
Presenting symptoms of common tropical illnesses

Disease	Fever	Rash	Myalgia	Arthralgia	Gastro-Intestinal	Jaundice	Spleno-Megaly	Hemorrhage	Neurologic	Respiratory	Headache
Malaria	XXX	—	XXX	X	XX	XX	XX	—	XX	X	XX
Dengue	XXX	X	XXX	X	XX	—	—	XX	XX	X	XX
ChikV	XXX	XX	XXX	XXX	XX	—	—	—	—	—	XX
Travelers' diarrhea	X	—	X	—	XXX	—	—	—	—	—	—

X: may be present; XX: probably present; XXX: definitively present.

TRAVELERS' DIARRHEA

Travelers' diarrhea (TD) is thought to occur in over 60% of individuals traveling from developed countries to less developed countries.[21] TD should be considered if an individual develops the passage of 3 or more loose stools in 24 hours.[22] Numerous etiologies exist for TD and are specific to region of travel.[23] The most common pathogens contributing to TD are strains of *Escherichia coli*: enterotoxigenic, enteroaggregative, and enteropathogenic. *E coli* incubation period is 1 to 4 days.[24] Gastrointestinal symptoms include diarrhea, abdominal cramps, and possibly fever and vomiting depending on the E coli stain. Diarrhea associated with *E coli* may produce bloody stools. All 3 strains of *E coli* are found in Haiti in addition to cholera.

Cholera had not been in Haiti for centuries but emerged after the 2010 earthquake. Cholera is an acute, diarrheal illness caused by the bacterium *Vibrio cholerae*.[25] Cholera produces watery stool but clinically is difficult to differentiate from other pathogens. Stool cultures remain the standard method of identifying the causing pathogen.[25]

E coli and cholera-induced TD are susceptible to azithromycin, which is safe for use in children. Azithromycin may be dosed 500 to 1000 mg daily for 1 to 3 days with pediatric dosing of 10 mg/kg/d for 3 days.[26] A fluoroquinolone such ciprofloxacin 500 mg 2 times daily for 3 days is an alternate drug choice in adults.[22] Aggressive oral rehydration will prevent severe illness, as many individuals with TD will suffer from mild-to-moderate dehydration.

Prophylaxis treatment for TD is not recommended at this time due to growing concern for antibiotic resistance.[22] Prevention of foodborne illness is recommended by following simple guidelines of eating boiled food and food that can be peeled. Travelers should not drink tap water or drinks that contain ice.

SUMMARY

Individuals traveling to Haiti are at risk for multiple topical illnesses that have similar presenting symptoms (**Table 4**). The assessment and care of travelers may be hindered by the health care provider's knowledge regarding the types of infectious disease individuals may encounter while traveling. Triage needs to occur rapidly by assessing a travel history. The CDC offers endless resources on identifying travel-related disease and clinical presentations with disease management. Identifying diseases that are prevalent in the traveled region will provide a starting point for care. Nurses need to ensure that a thorough history is taken regarding dates of travel, length of travel, exposure risk, timing of presenting symptoms, vaccinations prior to travel, and use of chemoprophylaxis.[27] Knowledge of potential exposure will allow for rapid care that may save individual lives if severe rapidly progressing disease is acquired.

REFERENCES

1. Freedman D, Weld L, Kozarsky P, et al. Spectrum of disease and relation to place of exposure among ill returned travelers. N Engl J Med 2006;345:119.
2. Bhatt S, Gething P, Brady O, et al. The global and burden of dengue. Nature 2013;496:504.
3. Dengue control. World Health Organization Web site. 2015. Available at: http://www.who.int/denguecontrol/en/. Accessed May 18, 2015.

4. World Health Organization and the Special Programme for Research and Training in Tropical Diseases. Dengue guidelines for diagnosis, treatment, prevention and control. Geneva (Switzerland): World Health Organization; 2009.
5. Immunizations, vaccines, and biologicals. World Health Organization Web site. 2014. Available at: http://www.who.int/immunization/diseases/dengue/en/. Accessed May 18, 2015.
6. Blacksell S. Commercial dengue rapid diagnostic tests for point-of-care application: recent evaluations and future needs? J Biomed Biotechnol 2012;2012:1–12.
7. Duong V, Ly S, Lorn Try P, et al. Clinical and virological factors influencing the performance of a NS1 antigen capture assay and potential use as a marker of dengue disease severity. PLoS Negl Trop Dis 2011;5:e1244.
8. Clinical assessment: Tourniquet test. Centers for Disease Control and Prevention Web site. Available at: http://www.cdc.gov/dengue/training/cme/ccm/page 73112.html. Accessed May 18, 2015.
9. Chuansumrit A, Tangnararatchakit K. Pathophysiology and management of dengue hemorrhagic fever. Transfus Altern Transfus Med 2006;8(Suppl 1):3–11.
10. Capeding MR, Tran NH, Hadinegoro SR, et al. Clinical efficacy and safety of a novel tetravalent dengue vaccine in healthy children in Asia: a phase 3, randomized observer-masked, placebo-controlled trial. Lancet 2014;384(9951):1358–65.
11. Chikungunya Fever. Centers for Disease Control and Prevention Web site. 2015. Available at: http://www.cdc.gov/chikungunya/. Accessed May 18, 2015.
12. Burt F, Rolph M, Rulli N, et al. Chikungunya: a re-emerging virus. Lancet 2012; 379:662.
13. Lakshmi V, Neeraja M, Subbalaxmi M, et al. Clinical features and molecular diagnosis of Chickungunya fever from South India. Clin Infect Dis 2008;46:1436.
14. Schilte C, Staikowsky F, Couderc T, et al. Chikungunya virus-associated long-term arthralgia: a 36-month prospective longitudinal study. PLoS Negl Trop Dis 2013;7:e2137.
15. Malaria. Centers for Disease Control and Prevention Web site. 2015. Available at: http://www.cdc.gov/malaria/index.html. Accessed May 20, 2015.
16. Cullen K, Arguin P, Centers for Disease Control and Prevention. Malaria surveillance—United Sates, 2012. MMWR Surveill Summ 2014;63:1.
17. Breman J. Clinical manifestation of malaria. UpToDate Web site. 2015. Available at: http://www.uptodate.com. Accessed May 15, 2015.
18. Severe malaria. Trop Med Int Health 2014;19(Suppl 1):7.
19. Yellow Book. Centers for Disease Control and Prevention. Available at: http://wwwnc.cdc.gov/travel/yellowbook/2014/chapter-3-infectious-diseases-related-to-travel/malaria. Accessed May 20, 2015.
20. Protection against mosquitoes, ticks, & other insects & arthropods. Centers for Disease Control and Prevention. 2013. Available at: http://wwwnc.cdc.gov/travel/yellowbook/2014/chapter-2-the-pre-travel-consultation/protection-against-mosquitoes-ticks-and-other-insects-and-arthropods. Accessed May 21, 2015.
21. Greenwood Z, Black J, Weld L, et al. Gastrointestinal infection among international travelers globally. J Travel Med 2008;15:221.
22. Nair D. Travelers' diarrhea: prevention, treatment, and post-trip evaluation. J Fam Pract 2013;63(7):356–61.
23. Shah N, DuPont H, Ramsey D. Global etiology of travelers' diarrhea: systematic review from 1973 to the present. Am J Trop Med Hyg 2009;80:609–14.
24. Foodborne outbreaks. Centers for Disease Control and Prevention Web site. 2013. Available at: http://www.cdc.gov/foodsafety/outbreaks/investigating-outbreaks/confirming_diagnosis.html. Accessed May 20, 2015.

25. Cholera. Centers for Disease Control and Prevention Web site. 2014. Available at: http://www.cdc.gov/cholera/general/index.html. Accessed May 20, 2015.

26. Kaushik J, Gupta P, Faridi M, et al. Single dose azithromycin versus ciprofloxacin for cholera in children: a randomized controlled trial. Indian Pediatr 2010;47: 309–15.

27. Wilson M. Evaluation of fever in the returning traveler. UpToDate. 2015. Available at: http://www.uptodate.com. Accessed May 15, 2015.

Pharmacology Update on Chronic Obstructive Pulmonary Disease, Rheumatoid Arthritis, and Major Depression

CrossMark

Deborah Weatherspoon, PhD, MSN, RN, CRNA[a,*],
Christopher A. Weatherspoon, APRN, MS, FNP-BC[b,c],
Brianna Abbott, BS[d]

KEYWORDS

- COPD • Breo Ellipta • Major depression • Brintellix • Rheumatoid arthritis • Xeljanz

KEY POINTS

- Breo Ellipta is a combination inhaled medication with fluticasone furoate and vilanterol indicated for use in patients with chronic obstructive pulmonary disease or asthma who are refractory to inhaled corticosteroid monotherapy.
- Brintellix (vortioxetine) is an immediate-release tablet for oral administration proven effective against depressive symptoms in both short-term and long-term scenarios.
- Xeljanz (tofacitinib) is the first of a unique class of oral kinase inhibitors to be approved by the Food and Drug Administration for the treatment of rheumatoid arthritis.

INTRODUCTION

Health care is a dynamic entity that is ever evolving. Chronic obstructive pulmonary disease (COPD), rheumatoid arthritis (RA), and major depression disorder (MDD) are frequently seen in primary care for treatment or as comorbidity to other health care issues. Although specialists may treat these disorders, it is important for the nurse practitioner (NP) to be familiar with new and current therapies that may affect other treatment plans. In addition, the NP must be knowledgeable and able to provide education on available therapies that patients inquire about. This is especially important

The authors have nothing to disclose.
[a] Core Faculty Leadership and Management Specialty College of Health Sciences, School of Nursing Graduate Program, Walden University, Washington Avenue South, Suite 900 Minneapolis, MN 55401, USA; [b] Veteran Affairs, Tennessee Valley Health System, Fort Campbell, KY, USA; [c] Contributing Faculty College of Health Sciences, School of Nursing Graduate Program, Walden University, Washington Avenue South, Suite 900 Minneapolis, MN 55401, USA; [d] College of Health Science, Bethel University, 325 Cherry Avenue, McKenzie, TN 38201, USA
* Corresponding author.
E-mail address: Deborah.Weatherspoon@Waldenu.edu

because use of the Internet, friends, or advertisements may leave the patient with inaccurate information. The purpose of this article is to review selected new pharmacologic treatments for COPD, MDD, and RA.

CHRONIC OBSTRUCTIVE PULMONARY DISEASE

The prevalence of COPD is steadily increasing despite leveling in Europe.[1] Previously considered a single disease, today COPD is defined as a broad syndrome that is not fully reversible.[2,3] This long-term lung disease, characterized by breathlessness, cough, and sputum production, limits activity and reduces the quality of life while increasing the incidence of premature death.[4] The World Health Organization reports that in 2012, more than 3 million people, or 6% of all deaths globally, are attributable to COPD.[5]

As the name implies, airway obstruction occurs and limits expiratory flow, resulting in air trapping, lung hyperinflation, and dyspnea. Pulmonary medications for COPD aim to decrease bronchial smooth muscle contraction, bronchial mucosal congestion and edema, airway inflammation, and secretions, thereby improving quality of life, slowing decline, and treating or preventing exacerbations.[6,7] In keeping with international recommendations, the severity of airway obstruction is based on the level of forced expiratory volume in 1 second percentage ($FEV_1\%$) predicted (**Table 1**).[8]

Patients with mild disease may respond to an inhaled short-acting beta agonist, for example, salbutamol or terbutaline, or a short-acting muscarinic antagonist, for example, ipratropium, to treat breathless and/or improve exercise limitation.[4] Although effective, beta-agonists have uncomfortable side effects of tremor and tachycardia. Anticholinergic agents improve FEV1 and reduce exacerbations.[6] Salbutamol has a faster onset of action, approximately 5 minutes compared with 30 to 60 minutes for ipratropium.[4,6]

The primary goal of pharmacologic treatment is to dilate the airways. Bronchodilators relieve breathlessness and are the cornerstone of treatment for patients with COPD. In mild-to-moderate patients ($FEV_1 \geq 50\%$ predicted) who are symptomatic or experience exacerbations, a long-acting beta2 agonist (LABA), for example, salmeterol or indacaterol, or a long-acting muscarinic antagonist, for example, tiotropium or glycopyrronium bromide, may be prescribed.[4,7]

Participants whose FEV_1 is less than 50% predicted may respond well to combination therapies of LABA/inhaled corticosteroids (ICS). Trials provide evidence that combination therapy improves quality of life and benefits lung function.[7,9] The National Institute for Health and Clinical Excellence provides an excellent decision model for treating COPD.[10] The Global Initiative for COPD also developed guidelines and

Table 1
2010 National Institute for Clinical Excellence guideline grading of severity of airflow obstruction

Severity	FEV_1 % Predicted
Stage 1—mild	$\geq 80^a$
Stage 2—moderate	50–79
Stage 3—severe 30–49	30–49
Stage 4—very severe	$<30^b$

Abbreviation: FEV_1, forced expiratory volume in 1 second.
  [a] Symptoms should be present to diagnose chronic obstructive pulmonary disease in people with mild airflow obstruction.
  [b] Or FEV_1 less than 50% with respiratory failure.

recommend a combination of an ICS and an LABA in patients with severe disease (stage III and IV) with frequent exacerbations.[8] Currently, there are 5 ICS/LABA combination products available,[11] as shown in **Table 2**.

The newest combination inhaler is Breo Ellipta (fluticasone furoate and vilanterol inhalation powder). The Food and Drug Administration (FDA) approved Breo Ellipta in May 2013 for the treatment and management of COPD.[10,12] Breo Ellipta is a combination inhaled medication with fluticasone furoate and vilanterol. ICSs and long-acting β2 agonists have been a mainstay in the treatment of COPD and asthma. Breo Ellipta is currently indicated for use only in patients with COPD or asthma who are refractory to ICS monotherapy; this indication is due to the class black box warning of using LABAs for the treatment of asthma.[13]

During clinical trials using patients with moderate to severe COPD, a statistically significant increase in FEV_1 was accomplished with all dosages of the medication.[14,15] With increased lung function and a decrease in exacerbations, this may equate to a significant improvement in overall quality of life.

Breo Ellipta has an advantage of single daily dosage compared with other combination medications, such as Advair, that require twice-daily dosage. The dosage for Breo Ellipta is once daily in a new proprietary device called Ellipta. This device, compared with the diskus device, was found to be preferable by patients with COPD for inhalation therapy.[16] The Ellipta device is scheduled for use with several other medications in the GlaxoSmithKline line up.[15]

Breo Ellipta is supplied in 100/25-μg and 200/25-μg dosages with initial treatment for COPD and asthma starting at 100/25 μg once daily. It is contraindicated in the primary treatment of status asthmaticus, acute episodes for COPD, or severe hypersensitivity to milk proteins. Warnings and precautions are similar to all ICS and LABA medications, with the most common adverse reactions to include nasopharyngitis (9%), oral candidiasis (5%), and headaches (7%). Use with caution if a patient is taking a cytochrome P450 3A4 inhibitor, such as ketoconazole, beta blockers, or diuretics, and use extreme caution when used concomitantly with monoamine oxidase inhibitors. Breo Ellipta is in pregnancy category C.[13]

An analysis of ICS/LABA combinations was found to have a class effect with regard to the prevention of COPD exacerbations. Although the preference for the Ellipta device[16] and the effectiveness of Breo Ellipta sound promising, no particular formulation is better than the other.[15]

Another consideration is the changing frame or definition for COPD. Traditionally, disease severity has been equated with the degree of airflow obstruction. However,

Table 2
Inhaled corticosteroid/long-acting beta2 agonist pharmaceuticals

Generic Name	Brand Name(s)	Manufacturer
Budesonide/formoterol (BUD/FM)	Symbicort	AstraZeneca, Wilmington, DE, USA
Fluticasone propionate/salmeterol (FP/SAL)	Advair, Seretide, Viani, Adoair, or Foxair	GlaxoSmithKline, Brentford, UK
Mometasone/formoterol (MF/FM)	Dulera or Zenhale	Merck, White House Station, NJ, USA
Beclomethasone dipropionate/formoterol (BDP/FM)	Fostair	Chiesi Ltd, Cheadle, UK
Fluticasone furoate/vilanterol (FF/VI)	Breo or Relvar Ellipta	GlaxoSmithKline

in recent years there has been an increasing recognition that COPD is not just a disease of the lungs, but has systemic manifestations; for example, depression, muscle wasting, and general fatigue.[9] Practitioners should keep these comorbidities in mind when patients present with additional symptoms to their COPD (**Box 1**).

MAJOR DEPRESSIVE DISORDER

Major depression is generally diagnosed when a persistent and unreactive low mood or sadness and/or loss of interest and pleasure are accompanied by a range of symptoms including appetite loss, insomnia, fatigue, loss of energy, poor concentration, psychomotor symptoms, inappropriate guilt, and morbid thoughts of death.[17] Debilitating effects of this condition include personal, social, and economic morbidity; loss of functioning; and productivity; in addition, it creates significant demands on service providers in terms of workload.[18,19] MDD has lifetime prevalence in the United States of 16.2%.[20]

Both pharmacologic and psychological interventions are effective for major depression. Antidepressant (AD) drugs are the mainstay of treatment in moderate to severe major depression and include many different agents.[19,21] A list of some current pharmacologic agents is provided in **Table 3**.

The development of selective serotonin reuptake inhibitors (SSRIs) has drastically improved the management of depression. Based on the amine hypothesis, selective inhibition of the reuptake of 5-HT receptors promotes functional increase in the activity of the central nervous system amine neurotransmitters norepinephrine, serotonin, and dopamine. During the past 20 years, AD prescription has dramatically risen in Western countries, mainly because of the increasing prescription of SSRIs and serotonin-noradrenaline reuptake inhibitors. SSRIs are generally more acceptable than tricyclic antidepressants, and there is evidence of similar efficacy.[19]

Although they are often a first-line choice, SSRIs have some undesirable effects. It may take weeks for SSRIs to reach therapeutic levels. In addition, there are some potential undesirable side effects, including decreased libido, retarded ejaculation, weight gain, insomnia, headaches, and nausea.

Considering what is new in pharmacologic management of depression, vortioxetine (Brintellix) appears to be a rising star. This relative newcomer to the antidepressants was FDA approved for the treatment of MDD in the fall of 2013.[22] Vortioxetine is a serotonin modulator and stimulator of the psychotropic class of chemical compounds known as bis-aryl-sulphanyl amines.[23] Vortioxetine is a novel multimodal compound for the treatment of MDD. It is a selective serotonin (5-HT) 3A and 5-HT7 receptor antagonist, 5-HT1B receptor partial agonist, 5-HT1A receptor agonist, and inhibitor of serotonin transporters.[22,24–26] The multiple mechanisms of action, which include

---

Box 1
Quick facts about breo ellipta

- Once-daily dosing
- Increases lung function and decreases exacerbations for patients with chronic obstructive pulmonary disease (COPD)
- Approved for patients with COPD and complicated asthma
- Side effects similar to other inhaled corticosteroid and long-acting beta2 agonist medications
- Starting dosage 100/25 μg

Table 3	
Antidepressant medications	
Antidepressant Medications Class	**Generic (Common Name Brand)**
Tricyclics (TCAs)	• Amitriptyline (Elavil) • Nortriptyline (Aventyl) • Doxepin (Sinequan) • Imipramine (Tofranil)
Monoamine oxidase inhibitors (MAOIs)	• Isocarboxazid (Marplan) • Phenelzine sulfate (Nardil) • Tranylcypromine sulfate (Parnate)
Selective serotonin reuptake inhibitors (SSRIs)	• Fluoxetine (Prozac) • Citalopram (Celexa) • Fluvoxamine (Luvox) • Sertraline (Zoloft) • Paroxetine (Paxil) • Escitalopram (Lexapro)
Serotonin-noradrenaline reuptake inhibitors (SNRIs)	• Venlafaxine (Effexor) • Duloxetine (Cymbalta)

serotonin reuptake inhibition and receptor activity modulation, affects several neurotransmitter pathways and increases the levels of noradrenaline, dopamine, acetylcholine, and histamine in the brain. These surges resulted in antidepressant properties, anxiolytic effects, and improvement of memory in rodent models.[23]

Vortioxetine is effective against depressive symptoms in both short-term and long-term scenarios. A meta-analysis of 7 randomized controlled trials demonstrated the efficacy of vortioxetine in reducing depression symptoms in adult patients with MDD.[22] A significant number of patients with MDD who were on vortioxetine therapy have achieved a greater than or equal to 50% depression symptom reduction from baseline based on both the Montgomery-Asberg Depression Rating Scale and the Hamilton Rating Scale for Depression.[22] The decrease in depression symptoms is intensified with an increase in the dose of vortioxetine. Furthermore, the efficacy of vortioxetine did not appear to decrease with long-term use; in 2 multicenter, open-label, flexible-dose extension studies, the efficacy of vortioxetine in the treatment of MDD was maintained for approximately 12 months.[27,28]

Vortioxetine is an immediate-release tablet for oral administration. The initial dosage is 10 mg per day with no regard to meals. The dosage is then increased to 20 mg per day as tolerated. Lower dosages should be considered for patients who do not tolerate the higher dosages. There is no contraindication for abrupt discontinued use; however, it is recommended that reduction to 10 mg per day for 1 week should be implemented if possible.[29]

Side effects reported include gastrointestinal disorders (nausea, diarrhea, dry mouth, constipation, vomiting, and flatulence), nervous system disorders (dizziness), psychiatric disorders (abnormal dreams), and skin and subcutaneous tissue disorders (pruritus). The most common adverse effects for vortioxetine were nausea, constipation, and vomiting.[29] Nausea was the most common adverse reaction and it generally occurred in the first week of therapy; however, 10% of patients continued to have nausea 6 to 8 weeks into therapy.[22]

Like many other antidepressant medications, vortioxetine carries a black box warning of the risk of increased suicidal thoughts and behaviors if used in children, adolescents, and young adults (age <25). It is a pregnancy category C. Currently vortioxetine is indicated for the treatment of MDD.[29] Further studies are in process to seek approval for the treatment of generalized anxiety disorder as well as the sexual functioning side effects of vortioxetine compared with SSRIs.

RHEUMATOID ARTHRITIS

RA is a systemic, autoimmune disease that causes chronic joint inflammation with periods of increased inflammation and remission. RA affects approximately 1.3 million adults in the United States.[30] The estimated burden of RA includes annual health care costs of $8.4 billion and total annual societal costs of $19.3 billion.

RA occurs most frequently in women and symptoms may appear earlier in life, between ages 30 and 60, compared with men. The exact cause of the disease is unknown; however, estrogen may be a factor due to the increased incidence in women. Cigarette smoking; occupational exposure to silica, wood, or asbestos; and certain infections are identified as risks and studies continue.

Although there is no cure for RA, a number of effective treatment options are available. Treatment for RA usually is initiated with nonbiologic disease-modifying antirheumatic drugs (DMARDs), such as leflunomide or methotrexate.[31,32] Treatment goals are to prevent or control joint damage and prevent loss of function. Pain control is a primary goal and includes several analgesics. For minor pain, acetaminophen may be effective. Nonsteroidal anti-inflammatory or cyclooxygenase-2 drugs relieve pain and reduce inflammation. Corticosteroids are often prescribed to treat acute symptoms; higher doses of corticosteroids require tapering before discontinuing.

The next line of treatment is DMARDs that reduce pain and inflammation and slow RA joint damage. DMARDs are prescribed as a monotherapy or in combination with other medication. In a systematic literature review of 30 randomized clinical trials, DMARDs as a monotherapy was compared with DMARDs in combination with methotrexate and found to be effective in patients with an inadequate response to conventional DMARDs.[33] One drawback is that DMARDs, such as methotrexate, may take weeks or even months to have an effect.[34]

Yet another category of medication for RA is that of biologics. These medications are prescribed in moderate to severe RA to slow progression of joint damage and to reduce signs and symptoms. Biologics are often used in combination with methotrexate or other DMARDs.

Patients with early RA who present with moderate or high disease activity, or who have an inadequate response to methotrexate monotherapy, or DMARD combination therapy, should be considered for biologic therapy with anti–tumor necrosis factor (TNF) or the non-TNF biologics abatacept or rituximab.[32] First-line biologic therapies are proven effective in slowing the progression of structural damage and improving the physical function of patients with moderate to severe RA.[32,35] Lack of response or loss of benefit warrants switching to a different biologic therapy, although little guidance exists as to which therapy is preferable to use as a second or subsequent agent (**Table 4**).[32]

Another concern for patients is that most biologics are administered by infusion or injection. The inconvenience of a clinic visit or even a dislike of needles may present a barrier to compliance. All biologics may increase the risk of infection or some cancers due to immune suppression. Patient education on the importance of treatment is needed to address these issues.

In November 2012, the FDA approved the use of an oral biologic, Xeljanz (tofacitinib) to treat adults with moderate to severe active RA.[36,37] Xeljanz, a pill taken twice daily,

Table 4
First-line biologic therapies

Generic	Common Name Brand
Abatacept	ORENCIA
Adalimumab	Humira
Certolizumab pegol	CIMZIA
Etanercept	Enbrel
Golimumab (in combination with methotrexate)	SIMPONI
Infliximab (in combination with methotrexate)	Remicade
Tocilizumab	ACTEMRA

works by blocking molecules called Janus kinases (JAK), enzymes that are important in the joint inflammation of RA.[36,37] JAKs mediate signaling by surface receptors for several important cytokines that are fundamental to the propagation of inflammation in RA. Tofacitinib prevents signaling of JAK enzymes and therefore interrupts important signal transduction of cytokines that contribute to the aberrant immune response in RA.

The safety and effectiveness of tofacitinib were evaluated in 7 clinical trials of adult patients with moderately to severely active RA. In all of the trials, patients treated with tofacitinib experienced improvement in clinical response and physical functioning compared with patients treated with placebo.[37–39] The use of tofacitinib was associated with an increased risk of serious infections, including opportunistic infections (infections that occur primarily when the immune system is suppressed), tuberculosis, cancers, and lymphoma. Tofacitinib carries a boxed warning regarding these safety risks. Tofacitinib treatment is also associated with increases in cholesterol and liver enzyme tests and decreases in blood counts. It is available only by prescription and is a pregnancy category C.

SUMMARY

This article presents a brief view of 3 distinct clinical conditions and an example of the most current therapies available. NPs may notice an increase in the incidence of adult patients diagnosed and receiving treatment for COPD and/or RA, as both of these diseases are chronic and frequently associated with an aging population. Although MDD may present in all ages as a primary diagnosis, it may also present as a comorbidity to chronic disease, especially diseases such as COPD and RA that interfere with quality of life. Although the information presented is not intended to be all inclusive, it does provide an overview of 3 relatively new pharmacologic agents that the NP may see patients presenting with in their practice.

REFERENCES

1. Lundback B, Bakke P, Ingebrigtsen T, et al. Chronic obstructive pulmonary disease. Eur Respir Monogr 2014;65:1–17.
2. Celli B, MacNee W. Standards for the diagnosis and treatment of patients with COPD: a summary of the ATS/ERS position paper. Eur Respir J 2004;23:932–46.
3. Vestbo J, Hurd SS, Agusti AG, et al. Global strategy for the diagnosis, management, and prevention of chronic obstructive pulmonary disease: GOLD executive summary. Am J Respir Crit Care Med 2013;187:347–65.
4. Hodson M, Sherrington R. Treating patients with chronic obstructive pulmonary disease. Nurs Stand 2014;29(9):50–8.

5. World Health Organization Web site. Chronic obstructive pulmonary disease (COPD). Available at: http://www.who.int/mediacentre/factsheets/fs315/en/. Accessed August 28, 2015.

6. Weatherspoon D, Weatherspoon C. Pulmonary problems. In: Foster JG, Prevost SE, editors. Advanced practice nursing of adults in acute care. Philadelphia: FA Davis; 2012. p. 398–444.

7. Kew KM, Dias S, Cates CJ. Long-acting inhaled therapy (beta-agonists, anticholinergics and steroids) for COPD: a network meta-analysis. Cochrane Database Syst Rev 2014;(3):CD010844.

8. Global Initiative for Obstructive Lung Disease (GOLD). Global strategy for the diagnosis, management, and prevention of chronic obstructive lung disease. Global Initiative for Obstructive Lung Disease (GOLD); 2011. Available at: http://www.goldcopd.org/guidelines-global-strategy-for-diagnosis-management.html. Accessed August 28, 2015.

9. Gruffydd-Jones K, Jones MM. NICE guidelines for chronic obstructive pulmonary disease: implications for primary care. Br J Gen Pract 2011;61(583):91–2.

10. Goldenberg MM. Pharmaceutical approval update. P T 2013;38(7):389–403.

11. National Institute for Health and Clinical Excellence 2010 guidelines: algorithm for inhaled pharmacotherapy in chronic obstructive pulmonary disease. Available at: http://www.ncbi.nlm.nih.gov/pmc/articles/PMC3026147/. Accessed August 28, 2015.

12. GlaxoSmithKline. Breo Ellipta, highlights of prescribing information. 2015. Available at: https://www.gsksource.com/pharma/content/dam/GlaxoSmithKline/US/en/Prescribing_Information/Breo_Ellipta/pdf/BREO-ELLIPTA-PI-MG.PDF. Accessed August 28, 2015.

13. Kerwin EM, Scott-Wilson C, Sanford L, et al. A randomised trial of fluticasone furoate/vilanterol (50/25 µg; 100/25 µg) on lung function in COPD. Respir Med 2013;107(12):2094.

14. GlaxoSmithKline. BREO™ ELLIPTA™ (fluticasone furoate/vilanterol inhalation powder) for treatment of chronic obstructive pulmonary disease NDA 204275. Available at: http://www.fda.gov/downloads/advisorycommittees/committees meetingmaterials/drugs/pulmonary-allergydrugsadvisorycommittee/ucm347931.pdf. Accessed August 28, 2015.

15. Oba Y, Lone NA. Comparative efficacy of inhaled corticosteroid and long-acting beta agonist combinations in preventing COPD exacerbations: a Bayesian network meta-analysis. Int J Chron Obstruct Pulmon Dis 2014;9:469.

16. U.S. National Institutes of Health. Diskus vs. ellipta device preference study in chronic obstructive pulmonary disease. ClinicalTrials.gov. 2014. NCT01868009. Available at: https://clinicaltrials.gov/ct2/show/results/NCT01868009?sect=X87056#outcome2. Accessed August 28, 2015.

17. National Institutes of Health. What is depression? Available at: http://www.nimh.nih.gov/health/topics/depression/index.shtml. Accessed August 28, 2015.

18. American Psychiatric Association. American Psychiatric Association practice guidelines for the treatment of psychiatric disorders: compendium 2006. American Psychiatric Association; 2006. Available at: http://psychiatryonline.org/pb/assets/raw/sitewide/practice_guidelines/guidelines/mdd.pdf. Accessed August 28, 2015.

19. National Institute for Clinical Excellence. Depression: management of depression in primary and secondary care—NICE guidance. London: National Institute for Clinical Excellence; 2010.

20. Beach SR, Whisman MA. Affective disorders. J Marital Fam Ther 2012;38(1):201–19.

21. Cipriani A, Purgato M, Furukawa TA, et al. Citalopram versus other anti-depressive agents for depression. Cochrane Database Syst Rev 2012;(7):CD006534.
22. Berhan A, Barker A. Vortioxetine in the treatment of adult patients with major depressive disorder: a meta-analysis of randomized double-blind controlled trials. BMC Psychiatry 2014;14:276.
23. Gibb A, Deeks ED. Vortioxetine: first global approval. Drugs 2014;74:135–45.
24. Bang-Andersen B, Ruhland T, Jørgensen M, et al. Discovery of 1-[2-(2,4-dime-thylphenylsulfanyl)phenyl]piperazine (Lu AA21004): a novel multimodal com-pound for the treatment of major depressive disorder. J Med Chem 2011;54(9): 3206–21.
25. Mork A, Pehrson A, Brennum LT, et al. Pharmacological effects of Lu AA21004: a novel multimodal compound for the treatment of major depressive disorder. J Pharmacol Exp Ther 2012;340:666–75.
26. Boulenger J, Loft H, Olsen CK. Efficacy and safety of vortioxetine (Lu AA21004), 15 and 20 mg/day: a randomized, double-blind, placebo-controlled, duloxetine-referenced study in the acute treatment of adult patients with major depressive disorder. Int Clin Psychopharmacol 2014;29(3):138–49.
27. Alam MY, Jacobsen PL, Chen Y, et al. Safety, tolerability, and efficacy of vortioxe-tine (Lu AA21004) in major depressive disorder: results of an open-label, flexible-dose, 52-week extension study. Int J Neuropsychopharmacol 2014;29:36–44.
28. Baldwin DS, Thomas H, Ioana F. Vortioxetine (Lu AA21004) in the long-term open-label treatment of major depressive disorder. Curr Med Res Opin 2012;28(10): 1717–24.
29. Brintellix. (n.d.). Available at: https://www.brintellixhcp.com/. Accessed May 28, 2015.
30. Helmick CG, Felson DT, Lawrence RC, et al. Estimates of the prevalence of arthritis and other rheumatic conditions in the United States. Part I. Arthritis Rheum 2008;58(1):15. Available at: http://onlinelibrary.wiley.com/doi/10.1002/art.23177/abstract. Accessed February 18, 2015.
31. Saag KG, Teng GG, Patkar NM, et al. American College of Rheumatology 2008 recommendations for the use of nonbiologic and biologic disease-modifying antirheumatic drugs in rheumatoid arthritis. Arthritis Rheum 2008;59(6):762–84. Available at: http://onlinelibrary.wiley.com/doi/10.1002/art.23721/abstract. Ac-cessed February 18, 2015.
32. Singh JA, Furst DE, Bharat A, et al. 2012 update of the 2008 American College of Rheumatology recommendations for the use of disease-modifying antirheumatic drugs and biologic agents in the treatment of rheumatoid arthritis. Arthritis Care Res (Hoboken) 2012;64(5):625–39. Available at: http://onlinelibrary.wiley.com/doi/10.1002/acr.21641/abstract. Accessed February 18, 2015.
33. Buckley F, Best JH, Dejonckheere F, et al. Comparative efficacy of novel disease-modifying antirheumatic drugs as monotherapy and in combination with metho-trexate in rheumatoid arthritis patients with an inadequate response to traditional DMARDS: a network meta-analysis. Rheumatology 2014;53(Suppl 1):i88–9. Avail-able at: http://www.ispor.org/research_pdfs/46/pdffiles/PMS5.pdf. Accessed August 28, 2015.
34. Smolen JS, Breedveld FC, Burmester GR, et al. Treating rheumatoid arthritis to target: 2014 update of the recommendations of an international task force. Ann Rheum Dis 2015. [Epub ahead of print].
35. Lie E, Fagerli KM, Mikkelsen K, et al. First-time prescriptions of biological disease-modifying antirheumatic drugs in rheumatoid arthritis, psoriatic arthritis

and axial spondyloarthritis 2002–2011: data from the NOR-DMARD register. Ann Rheum Dis 2014;73:1905–6.

36. U.S. Department of Health & Human Services. FDA approves Xeljanz for rheumatoid arthritis. Available at: http://www.drugs.com/newdrugs/fda-approves-xeljanz-rheumatoid-arthritis-3558.html. Accessed August 28, 2015.

37. Traynor K. FDA approves tofacitinib for rheumatoid arthritis. Am J Health Syst Pharm 2012;69:2120.

38. van Vollenhoven RF, Fleischmann R, Cohen S, et al. Tofacitinib or adalimumab versus placebo in rheumatoid arthritis. N Engl J Med 2012;367:508–19.

39. van Vollenhoven RF. Small molecular compounds in development for rheumatoid arthritis. Curr Opin Rheumatol 2013;25:391–7.

Implementing a Program for Ultrasound-Guided Peripheral Venous Access

Training, Policy and Procedure Development, Protocol Use, Competency, and Skill Tracking

Richard P. Laksonen Jr, MSN, APRN, NP-C, NRP[a],*,
Nanci K. Gasiewicz, DNP, RN, CNE[b]

KEYWORDS

- Ultrasound guided • Intravenous access • Competency • Protocol

KEY POINTS

- Ultrasound-guided peripheral venous access provides a safe alternative to traditional methods of peripheral vascular access.
- When visualization of peripheral vasculature is poor, ultrasound-guided peripheral intravenous access provides a safe method for administration of medications, intravenous fluids and blood products.
- Although vasculopathies and chronic medical conditions contribute to difficult peripheral intravenous access, obesity is the most common cause for poor visualization and palpation of veins.
- Ultrasound-guided peripheral intravenous access bridges the practice gap between traditional methods of peripheral intravenous access and central venous access in adult patient with difficult peripheral intravenous access.
- This article presents a competency-based training program, policy, procedure, protocol and tracking system for training in the use of ultrasound-guided peripheral intravenous access (UGPIVA).

INTRODUCTION

For most hospitalized patients, peripheral intravenous (IV) access is needed to administer fluids, blood products, and potentially lifesaving medications.[1] When peripheral IV access is established in a timely fashion, patient outcomes are optimized.

The authors have nothing to disclose.
[a] Family Medicine, United States Air Force, 5th Medical Operations Squadron, 5th Medical Group, 5th Bomb Wing, Minot Air Force Base, Minot AFB, ND 58705, USA; [b] School of Nursing, Northern Michigan University, 1401 Presque Isle Avenue, Marquette, MI 49855, USA
* Corresponding author.
E-mail address: Richard.laksonen.1@us.af.mil

Nurs Clin N Am 50 (2015) 771–785
http://dx.doi.org/10.1016/j.cnur.2015.07.010
0029-6465/15/$ – see front matter © 2015 Elsevier Inc. All rights reserved.

nursing.theclinics.com

However, traditional methods for obtaining peripheral IV access are sometimes unsuccessful.

Traditional nursing approaches to peripheral IV access focus on the palpation/visualization technique. With this technique, nurses rely on being able to see or feel a suitable vein for peripheral cannulation. Often, patients do not have visible or palpable veins suitable for cannulation. Multiple factors, such as the age of the patient, dehydration, small or fragile veins, obesity, and a history of IV drug abuse, present particularly challenging situations for securing peripheral IV access.[2,3]

Significance

Multiple peripheral IV access attempts can increase a patient's anxiety, increase the overall procedural pain, increase the risk for infection, and most importantly delay vital treatment.[2(p199)] The Infusion Nurses Society recommends that patients undergo only 2 traditional percutaneous venipunctures before using other methods for establishing peripheral IV access.[4] If peripheral IV cannulation remains unsuccessful, an alternate route must be found.

Background

When peripheral IV cannulation is unsuccessful, central venous access may be deemed necessary and is usually performed by physicians because of the risk of serious complications such as pneumothorax, malpositioning of the cannula, local tissue damage, corresponding arterial punctures, or cardiac dysrhythmias.[5,6] Physician ability to provide timely central venous access can be difficult as they are often coordinating care for multiple patients at any given time. In addition, the risks of central venous access often outweigh the benefits when used in the non–critically ill patient population.

Real-time ultrasound guidance for establishment of central venous cannulation has been studied and used for the last 30 years. The safety of real-time ultrasound guidance has led the Agency for Healthcare Research and Quality to recommend it for all central venous access.[7] However, unless a patient requires particular medications that must be administered through a central catheter, or if central fluid monitoring must be documented, peripheral IV access is the preferred route because of ease of access and reduced risk of complications.[8]

Therefore, a practice gap exists between traditional methods of peripheral venous access and ultrasound-guided central venous access. Ultrasound-guided peripheral intravenous access (UGPIVA) provides a safe and reliable means of bridging this practice gap.

UGPIVA uses a live feed ultrasound screen that documents peripheral venous cannulation from skin puncture through venipuncture via direct visualization on an ultrasound monitor for the health care provider performing the skill in real time. This article presents a competency-based training program, policy, procedure, protocol, and tracking system for training registered nurses (RNs) in the skill and use of UGPIVA in adult patients.

REVIEW OF LITERATURE

In patients who present with difficult peripheral IV access, UGPIVA is more successful than traditional peripheral IV access techniques, requires less time, decreases the amount of percutaneous punctures, and improves patient satisfaction.[7(p458)] UGPIVA uses the same ultrasonographic technique that central venous access has used for 30 years. There is a low risk of patient complications associated with UGPIVA, and complications are usually limited to local events, such as phlebitis, pain, and irritation.[9]

A nurse-driven study of a UGPIVA program in an emergency department found that UGPIVA expedited treatment and disposition in the emergency department and was successful in 90% to 98% of the patients that it was used on.[10] The UGPIVA program referenced in this study has been in place since 2009, with continued favorable outcomes.[10(p49)]

Definitions

Difficult peripheral IV access across the literature is defined as 2 or 3 unsuccessful peripheral IV access attempts or a history of difficult peripheral IV access.[11,12]

UGPIVA is defined as the use of an ultrasound probe to identify vasculature in a patient's arm, select a viable vein for cannulation, and directly visualize a peripheral IV catheter entering the vein.

Ultrasound probes are wandlike devices placed on the patients' skin to assist with visualization of vasculature. Vasculature is viewed on a monitor screen. Linear ultrasound probes, which are most often used for UGPIVA, are those with a frequency of 5 to 13 MHz.[13]

Patients are defined as adults, 18 years and older, who require peripheral IV access. Although UGPIVA can be performed in the pediatric population, there is scant literature that specifically addresses the use of UGPIVA in the pediatric population.

Patient Characteristics

Patients present with a variety of reasons that make peripheral IV access difficult. Although vasculopathies and chronic medical conditions are related to difficult peripheral IV access, obesity is likely the most common difficulty identified as it completely removes the method of visualization and palpation traditionally used for peripheral IV access. Rates of obesity in the United States are increasing, and as a result, the subset of patients requiring alternative methods of venous access is increasing.[12(p475)]

Educational Characteristics

The literature reflects several studies using a wide variety of health care providers to establish UGPIVA. Training for physicians varies widely from a 30-minute purely didactic session to a 30-minute workshop followed by 60 minutes of skills application time to a 2-day course in UGPIVA with an additional 2-week refresher rotation in ultrasonography within the first year of physician residency training.[14–16] Nursing and emergency medical technician (EMT) training ranges from a 45- to 60-minute lecture and skills session to an 8-hour class split between lecture and skills learning.[17,18]

Training programs provide skills education using a phantom gel model to demonstrate visual representation of tissue types and vascular structures. The literature does not demonstrate a preference of one training program over another but rather supports a variety of teaching and learning techniques for mastery of UGPIVA.[17(p404),19] These techniques are discussed further under Ultrasound Techniques and Success Rates.

Operator Characteristics

The literature supports UGPIVA performed by physicians and nonphysicians as a safe and effective method to establish UGPIVA.[7(p460),20] Registered nurses and emergency medical technicians (EMTs) are referred to as nonphysicians throughout the remainder of this article.

Ultrasound Techniques

Various techniques have been used in UGPIVA. Ultrasound guidance provides real-time 2-dimensional images of underlying tissue and vasculature so the health care provider can readily and reliably obtain peripheral IV access.[21]

There are several ways to obtain ultrasonographic images. Use of ultrasound for the establishment of peripheral IV access was first found in the literature in 1999.[11(p712)] Before this, ultrasound-guided cannulation was reserved for use in central venous access.

In early studies of UGPIVA, a 2-provider technique was used in which one physician held a linear probe on the patients arm while the other provider performed the peripheral venipuncture.[11(p713)] Although the 2-person technique is convenient, the actual patient care environment in which UGPIVA is indicated often does not support the 2-person technique. Therefore, UGPIVA using a 1-person technique must be considered.

With the 1-person technique, the practitioner holds the ultrasound probe in the nondominant hand and places it on the arm of the patient for ultrasonographic analysis, then uses the dominant hand for venipuncture. In a study comparing techniques, no statistically significant difference was found in outcomes between UGPIVA using 1-operator and 2-operator techniques.[22]

Image analysis may use 1 of 2 ultrasound probe orientations, either perpendicular to the vessel (transverse/short axis) or directly over the vessel (longitudinal/long axis). Novice ultrasonographers usually obtain vascular access quicker using the transverse approach/short axis; however, the longitudinal/long-axis approach can enable the provider to visualize the needle entering the vessel in its entirety.[14(p1310)] In the longitudinal/long-axis approach, if a catheter was moving against an obstruction within the vessel, a valve, for example, it can be redirected under radiographic visualization.

Although much of the research uses the transverse/short-axis approach, the more experienced physician and nonphysician providers use the transverse/short-axis approach for initial visualization of the vein, then rotate the probe 90° into the longitudinal/long-axis orientation for full-vessel imaging.[13(pe39),18(p354),23] A study comparing success rates between the 2 ultrasound probe orientations found that differences in success rates were marginal, although fewer complications or inadvertent damage to adjacent structures in the upper arm were noted while using the longitudinal/long-axis approach.[24,25]

Any vessel that may be visualized with ease under a linear ultrasound probe may be cannulated using ultrasound guidance. The use of the brachial and basilic veins for cannulation is most common, as these are large vessels, with few convolutions or obstructions.[11(p714)]

Success Rates

Table 1 discusses UGPIVA success rates, number of providers, methodology, and physician versus nonphysician providers from a variety of studies.[3(p1362), 7(p460), 9(p498, 499), 11(p713), 15(p327), 17(p403, 404), 21(p856), 22(p434), 24(p1301), 26–31] After UGPIVA proficiency was achieved, perceptions of patients as being very hard to gain peripheral IV access went from 80% with traditional peripheral IV access methods to 11% with use of UGPIVA.[32]

Most of the literature reviewed supports use of UGPIVA. However, in a study conducted by anesthesia personnel, there was no difference in success rates of traditional peripheral IV access methods when compared with UGPIVA.[26(p213)] The success rates

Table 1
UGPIVA data

Author	Success Rate (%)	Control (%)	Probe Orientation	Provider Level	1- or 2-Person Technique
Aponte et al,[26] 2007	74	—	Transverse	Non-MD	1
Bauman et al,[27] 2009	80.5	70.6	Transverse	Non-MD	1
Brannam et al,[3] 2004	87	—	NA	Non-MD	1
Chinnock et al,[17] 2007	63	—	Transverse	Non-MD	1 or 2
Constantino et al,[7] 2005	97	33	Transverse	MD	2
Darvish et al,[28] 2011	NA	—	Transverse	Non-MD	1
Gregg et al,[29] 2010	99	—	Transverse	MD	1
Keyes et al,[11] 1999	91	—	Transverse	MD	2
Mahler et al,[15] 2010	96	—	Transverse	MD	1
Panebianco et al,[24] 2009	90	—	Transverse or Longitudinal	MD	1
Resnick et al,[30] 2008	73	—	Transverse or Longitudinal	MD and non-MD	1
Rose et al,[22] 2008	75	—	Transverse	MD	1 vs 2
Schoenfeld et al,[9] 2011	78.5	—	Transverse or Longitudinal	Non-MD	1
Walker,[21] 2009	97	—	Transverse	Non-MD	1
White et al,[31] 2010	96.9	—	NA	Non-MD	1

Abbreviations: MD, medical doctor; NA, not applicable.
  Data from Refs.[3,7,9,11,15,17,21,22,24(p1301),26–31]

between traditional methods of peripheral IV access and UGPIVA may have been affected by the population studied, as this was a sample of convenience in the preoperative setting and not identified as experiencing any difficulty with peripheral IV access.

A study done in an intensive care unit analyzed 2 interesting concepts, (1) overall success rates of the procedure and (2) discontinuation of central venous access devices, and as **Table 1** indicates, there was a 99% success rate with UGPIVA.[29(p517)] In addition, this study revealed that 40 central lines were discontinued and 34 central lines were completely avoided because UGPIVA was successfully used as a viable alternative to central venous cannulation.[29(p518)]

Ultrasound guidance enables visualization of veins not apparent on physical examination, resulting in fewer needle sticks, more rapid cannulation, and higher levels of patient satisfaction among patients experiencing difficult IV access.[7(p458),11(p712),19(p37)]

Learning ultrasound-guided techniques is easy, especially for providers who are proficient in placing standard venous access catheters.[13(pe39, e40),23(p126)]

Overall, the literature supports use of UGPIVA in adult patients experiencing difficulty with traditional methods of peripheral IV access. Although UGPIVA requires training sessions, it can be performed by physicians and nonphysicians using several techniques, while also improving successful peripheral IV access rates and patient satisfaction.

METHODOLOGY

Review of the literature supports UGPIVA as a viable method of peripheral IV access among patients experiencing difficulty with traditional methods of peripheral IV access, thus bridging the practice gap between traditional peripheral IV access methods and central venous access in patients. A competency-based training program, policy, procedure, protocol, and tracking system for training RNs in the skill and use of UGPIVA are presented here.

Policy and Procedure

As with any nursing skill or training program, a policy and procedure is developed and adopted to ensure consistency and quality of training and skill application. **Box 1** depicts a generic policy defining UGPIVA and its uses. **Box 2** illustrates a procedure outlining the necessary steps for use of UGPIVA.

Protocol

To better facilitate decision making, **Fig. 1** delineates a difficult venous access protocol. This protocol was developed using a flow process similar to algorithms used in various certification programs (ie, American Heart Association Advanced Cardiac Life Support). Using the protocol alleviates any gap in care during the decision-making process for use of UGPIVA in patients with difficult peripheral IV access. In time, the protocol will become a standard of care for UGPIVA. The UGPIVA protocol should be revised as needed based on current best practices found in the literature and patient outcomes, inclusive of patient satisfaction with the UGPIVA experience.

Training

The most time-consuming component of UGPIVA is development of training materials and program (competency) implementation. Because of lessons learned from previous program implementations, the training sessions were streamlined to include didactic content and skill practice in a combined 2-hour session. After the training session, the trainer remains on site to proctor UGPIVA on live patients with the newly UGPIVA-trained nurses. Owing to the unpredictability of patients with difficult peripheral venous access, healthy patients are used for initial live-patient UGPIVA. The UGPIVA trainer is an RN experienced in UGPIVA and, if available, an emergency department physician skilled in UGPIVA.

Training is repeated over the course of multiple days, with overlapping shift schedules. Program attendees include full-time and regular part-time RNs. Progression from one phase of training to the next does not occur until the student verbalizes comfort and has no further questions for the instructor.

Departmental nurse managers and assistant nurse managers should attend training sessions to serve as departmental UGPIVA advocates. These departmental-level nurse leaders usually work full time and do not carry a full patient

Box 1
Ultrasound-guided peripheral intravenous access policy

Scope: Registered Nurses

Physician order: Not required

Definition
UGPIVA uses a live feed ultrasound screen that documents peripheral intravenous (IV) cannulation from skin puncture through venipuncture via direct visualization on an ultrasound monitor for the health care provider performing the skill in real time. UGPIVA fills a gap in patient care between traditional peripheral IV access methods of vein visualization and/or palpation and ultrasound-guided or blind central venous access. This policy is for the establishment of peripheral IV access in patients with difficult access using UGPIVA in a safe manner.

Purpose
UGPIVA is used for identification of vasculature and successful placement of peripheral IV catheters in adult patients with difficult peripheral IV access. These patients are those

- Who require IV access to administer medications, fluids, and/or blood products that do not require central venous access
- Who have peripheral vasculature that is difficult to visualize and/or palpate
- Who have undergone 2 unsuccessful traditional visualization and/or palpation peripheral IV access attempts
- Who are otherwise poor candidates for additional peripheral vascular access methods (feet, mammary veins, external jugular veins, intraosseous devices)
- Who are otherwise not candidates for central venous access

Qualifications
UGPIVA is an advanced skill that requires additional training beyond traditional visualization and/or palpation techniques. A registered nurse is required to attend education and skill training and demonstrate validated competency in use of UGPIVA techniques that include

Initial training

- Initial didactic training that covers vessel anatomy, ultrasound science, UGPIVA approach techniques, review of UGPIVA policy, procedure, protocol, competency checklist, and access log
- Completion of the UGPIVA quiz
- Initial skills training with ultrasound machine, phantom gel model, and, if available, vessel identification on live patient volunteers.
- Three successful live-patient UGPIVA catheter insertions proctored by a UGPIVA facilitator

Annual recertification

- Four documented successful UGPIVA catheter insertions annually
  or
- Completion of the initial UGPIVA training module annually

UGPIVA should not be used if
- Physician states a contraindication
- Chemotherapeutic agent infusion is intended
- Continuous irritant or vesicant infusion is intended
- Pressure injections (ie, for contrast computed tomographic scans) are intended

Courtesy of R. Laksonen Jr, MSN, APRN, NP-C, NRP, Minot AFB, ND.

Box 2
Ultrasound-guided peripheral intravenous line access procedure

Procedure: Ultrasound-guided peripheral intravenous line access (UGPIVA)	Procedure No.:
Distribution:	Effective date:
Authorized by:	Revision date:

Knowledge: This procedure requires advanced competency.

Purpose: Placing peripheral intravenous lines by ultrasound in a safe practice

Equipment: Ultrasound with high-frequency (linear) probe, ultrasound gel, hospital standard IV start equipment

Providers: RNs certified through training program to include ultrasound-guided IV education course and module, as well as 5 observed gel phantom simulator attempts and 3 experienced ultrasound RN or physician-observed actual patient ultrasound-guided IV starts

Competencies: Nurses must document 4 successful ultrasound-guided IV insertions every calendar year. Each RN is accountable to keep records to maintain competency on the provided documentation form

Procedure	Point of Emphasis
Patient must be 18 years or older to perform procedure	A physician order is needed for patients younger than 15 years, with emphasis on predicted difficult starts
1. Explain the procedure to the patient and wash hands.	—
2. Disinfect the ultrasound probe with antimicrobial wipe.	—
3. Plug in ultrasound.	—
4. Apply tourniquet to proximal upper arm.	A blood pressure cuff may be substituted for patients with hypotension.
5. Adjust gain and depth of ultrasound view.	—
6. Identify brachial vessels 10 cm distal to 10 cm proximal to antecubital fossae. Identify cephalic vessel on the contralateral aspect of the arm 10 cm proximal and distal.	Use the largest vessel visualized.
7. Confirm identity as vein by compressing flat and absence of color Doppler pulsations.	Pulsatile motion on color Doppler and the inability to compress the vessel indicate arterial blood flow.
8. Switch from color mode back to 2-dimensional mode for maximum clarity.	—
9. Confirm that 0.4-cm-diameter or larger veins are within 1.5 cm of skin surface.	—
10. Confirm that vein course is sufficiently linear to insert the catheter.	—
11. Sterilize site as per routine peripheral IV protocol.	—
12. Apply ultrasound gel from ultrasound cart to probe head.	—
13. Directly observe needle enter the vein in a transverse orientation.	—
14. Place ultrasound probe in a safe location.	—
15. Advance the catheter and secure as per routine peripheral IV protocol.	Blood draw per hospital policy may occur at this point. Flush catheter with saline per protocol.
16. Disinfect the ultrasound probe with antimicrobial wipe.	—

Courtesy of R. Laksonen Jr, MSN, APRN, NP-C, NRP, Minot AFB, ND.

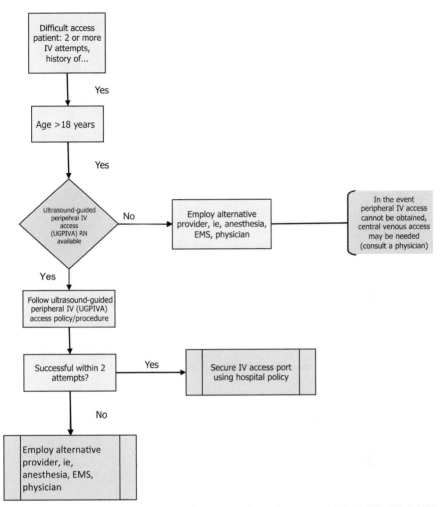

Fig. 1. Difficult venous access protocol. (*Courtesy of* R. Laksonen Jr, MSN, APRN, NP-C, NRP, Minot AFB, ND.)

care load, thus allowing them to assist with patient care, including UGPIVA. UGPIVA advocates maintain skill competence and serve as proctors for live-patient UGPIVA procedures.

Although the literature does not address any specifics related to individual training programs, a PowerPoint training module was developed to illustrate the most important topics regarding UGPIVA. Lecture topics include vessel anatomy, ultrasound science, and approach techniques. In addition, the UGPIVA policy, procedure, and protocol are also reviewed with students.

Presentation of the didactic portion of the training is designed to take approximately 1 hour, after which each student completes a 10-question quiz (**Box 3**). The quiz is not graded, and each answer is reviewed with students for teaching-learning value. There is no minimum quiz score needed to pass the didactic portion of UGPIVA training. Following didactic content, students are asked to demonstrate use of the ultrasound machine.

Box 3
Ultrasound-guided IV access quiz

Name:

Multiple choice: For each of the following questions, circle the letter of the answer that best answers the question.

1. Ultrasound-guided IV access can be used for
   A. Adult patients
   B. Neonatal patients
   C. Pediatric patients
   D. All of the above

2. The best vessel for ultrasound-guided IV access is
   A. Cephalic vein
   B. Brachial artery
   C. Basilic vein
   D. Median antecubital vein

True or False: For each statement, circle True or False.

True	False	1. Difficult access patients are candidates for ultrasound-guided IV access
True	False	2. Arteries appear as compressible black circles on the ultrasound screen
True	False	3. You do not have to clean the patients arm before placing an ultrasound IV
True	False	4. You use your dominant hand to hold the ultrasound probe
True	False	5. Veins appear as brightly colored pulsatile structures under color Doppler

3. The probe used for ultrasound-guided IV access is called the...probe
   A. Linear
   B. Rectal
   C. Big
   D. Low frequency

4. Which of the following medical conditions causes difficult IV access in patients?
   A. Obesity
   B. Renal failure
   C. IV drug use
   D. All of the above

5. The easiest way to view a vessel using ultrasound is the
   A. Transverse view
   B. Longitudinal view

Courtesy of R. Laksonen Jr, MSN, APRN, NP-C, NRP, Minot AFB, ND.

After use of the ultrasound machine has been mastered, students are asked to demonstrate vessel identification on both the phantom gel model and fellow students attending the training program. Because the transverse (short-axis) view has proved more effective for novice ultrasonographers, this is the technique used during initial training.[14(p1309–10)] Specific concepts emphasized during vessel identification are vessel tracking, type of vessel (vein vs artery), use of the Doppler function, additional tissue identification, and vessel selection.

As students become proficient in identification of vasculature, they are asked to practice a minimum of 5 successful live-practice UGPIVA procedures on the phantom gel model. The live-practice procedures are completed using the UGPIVA procedure in its entirety to ensure student familiarity with all components of the skill/procedure.

Once the student has demonstrated 5 successful UGPIVA procedures on the phantom gel model, the classroom-based training is complete.

Competency

Competency for independent use of UGPIVA requires the following:

- Five completed phantom gel model procedures
- Three successful proctored live-patient procedures
- Four successful UGPIVA procedures annually
- Documentation of UGPIVA procedures on UGPIVA tracking log

In the event students do not maintain UGPIVA proficiency, attendance at another UGPIVA training session is required, followed by 3 proctored UGPIVA procedures on live patients. Students who complete a minimum of 4 UGPIVA procedures annually are considered competent and not required to attend any additional training.

The didactic and skills application components of UGPIVA competency are tracked with use of a UGPIVA competency checklist (**Fig. 2**) and log (**Table 2**).

DISCUSSION
Limitations

An exhaustive literature review demonstrated that UGPIVA is a feasible skill to use in patients with difficult peripheral IV access. However, the literature review did not

Lecture Based Training

☐ Anatomy Review

☐ Ultrasound Machine

☐ Ultrasound Techniques

Instructor/Date_____

Practical Training

☐ Vessel Identification on Gel

☐ Vessel Identification on Partner

☐ Technique Demonstration on Gel (Must complete 5 successful catheter insertions)

Instructor/Date_____

Live Patient Ultrasound IV Starts

☐ Date: _____   Proctor:_____

☐ Date: _____   Proctor:_____

☐ Date: _____   Proctor:_____

Registered Nurse Name: _____

Registered Nurse Signature: _____

Fig. 2. Ultrasound-guided IV access competency checklist. (*Courtesy of* R. Laksonen Jr, MSN, APRN, NP-C, NRP, Minot AFB, ND.)

Table 2 Ultrasound-guided peripheral IV access log							
Date	Patient ID#	RN/MD Name	Site	Traditional (#)	UGPIVA (#)	Reason for Difficult Access	Successful? Comments

Courtesy of R. Laksonen Jr, MSN, APRN, NP-C, NRP, Minot AFB, ND.

contain any large, well-controlled trials examining each aspect of UGPIVA systematically.

Pediatric patients present a unique situation with traditional visualization and/or palpation techniques for peripheral IV access. Owing to lack of a large subcutaneous fat layer and well-developed muscular tissue, the pediatric population presents a particular challenge for UGPIVA, which relies on tissue differentiation for vasculature visualization. This aspect would inherently drive UGPIVA success rates lower in pediatric patients than in adult patients. A prospective, observational study of a convenience sample comparing peripheral IV access using the traditional visualization and/or palpation technique with UGPIVA in pediatric patients from July 2006 to February 2007 revealed a success rate of 42% for UGPIVA versus 38% using traditional visualization and/or palpation.[33] Both these success rates are considerably lower than those in comparable studies done in adults.

The absence of a dedicated UGPIVA advocate may prove problematic for ongoing success of UGPIVA programs. Experience demonstrates that UGPIVA programs flounder when an identified program advocate is not consistently present in the area or department where UGPIVA is used.

Start-up costs for UGPIVA can be considerable. The cost of ultrasound machines range between $15,000 for a reconditioned model to $35,000 for a new model. In addition, the phantom gel training models range in price from $359 to $429.[18(p355)] The remainder of the equipment needed for UGPIVA should be readily available, as it does not differ from standard IV therapy equipment.

Implications and Recommendations

Large, well-controlled trials examining every aspect of UGPIVA should be considered. In addition, translational research and best practice implementation should include UGPIVA procedures performed on actual patients and their relationship to provider confidence with skill competency.

It is essential to have designated UGPIVA advocates serve as proctors for those learning the UGPIVA procedure. Loss of trained UGPIVA advocates was the primary reason for program failure. Ideally, UGPIVA advocates have a desire to learn, use, and maintain proficiency with the skill to become a resource person and mentor for the others learning UGPIVA. Comparative analysis of programs using UGPIVA nurse advocates and those that do not could be done to test this assumption.

The skill must be documented and tracked just as traditional peripheral IV insertions. To identify measurable outcomes and determine the success of a UGPIVA training program, UGPIVA site survivability ideally should be equal or surpass that for traditional peripheral IV access sites. Potential complications found with peripheral IV insertions, such as infection, inflammation, phlebitis, extravasation, and infiltration, should be tracked and compared with those of UGPIVA procedures. In addition, details of serious UGPIVA insertion-related complications, such as nerve irritation, hematoma formation, and arterial puncture, should be accurately and appropriately documented and reported to providers and UGPIVA program coordinators.

Patient comfort and satisfaction with the UGPIVA procedure can also serve as indicators of program success.[31(p188)] Using outcome data can provide valuable quality assurance information for traditional peripheral IV access versus UGPIVA and ensure utilization of the most optimal peripheral IV access approach for patients. Qualitative analysis of patient experience regarding UGPIVA is warranted to ensure that subjective satisfaction ratings are paired well with objective success patterns.

When UGPIVA is used in the noncritically ill patient as a secondary option, it is advisable to assess subjective patient experience, as this can contribute to overall patient experience during hospitalization, and it is important to ensure a high level of patient satisfaction. If there is no positive correlation between patient satisfaction and UGPIVA use, alternate peripheral IV access methods should be explored.

SUMMARY

UGPIVA surpasses the traditional method of peripheral IV access both subjectively from the patient perspective and objectively through ease and success of peripheral IV access. The current best practices found in the literature also support use of UGPIVA. Thus, UGPIVA is a useful addition to the current skill set of those charged with securing peripheral IV access in adult patients.

A competency-based training program, policy, procedure, protocol, and tracking system for training RNs in the skill and use of UGPIVA has been developed and presented here. However, dedicated UGPIVA advocates and proctors are an essential part of program sustainability.

UGPIVA bridges the practice gap between traditional methods of peripheral IV access and central venous access in adult patients with difficult peripheral IV access. However, to ensure continued best practices and optimal patient outcomes, additional well-controlled research is needed to examine each aspect of UGPIVA systematically to further validate what has been anecdotally supported to this point.

REFERENCES

1. Neumar RW, Otto CW, Link MS, et al. Part 8: adult advanced cardiovascular life support: 2010 American Heart Association guidelines for cardiopulmonary resuscitation and emergency cardiovascular care. Circulation 2010;122(18 Suppl 3): S729–67.
2. Walsh G. Difficult peripheral venous access: recognizing and managing the patient at risk. J Assoc Vasc Access 2008;13(4):198–203.
3. Brannam L, Blaivas M, Lyon M, et al. Emergency nurses' utilization of ultrasound guidance for placement of peripheral intravenous lines in difficult-access patients. Acad Emerg Med 2004;11(12):1361–3.
4. Alexander M. Infusion nursing standards of practice. J Infus Nurs 2011;34(1S): S1–109. Available at: http://www.ins1.org/.
5. LeDonne J. Complications of central venous catheterization. J Am Coll Surg 2007;205:517.
6. Crowley M, Brim C, Proehl J, et al. Emergency nursing resource: difficult intravenous access. J Emerg Nurs 2012;38(4):335–43.

7. Costantino TG, Parikh AK, Satz WA, et al. Ultrasonography-guided peripheral intravenous access versus traditional approaches in patients with difficult intravenous access. Ann Emerg Med 2005;46(5):456–61.

8. Reynolds BR, Watson GA. Resuscitation from hemorrhagic shock. In: Tisherman SA, Forsythe RM, editors. Trauma intensive care. New York: Oxford University Press; 2013. p. 63–72.

9. Schoenfeld E, Boniface K, Shokoohi H. ED technicians can successfully place ultrasound-guided intravenous catheters in patients with poor vascular access. Am J Emerg Med 2011;29(5):496–501.

10. Moore C. An emergency department nurse-driven ultrasound-guided peripheral intravenous line program. J Assoc Vasc Access 2013;18(1):45–51.

11. Keyes LE, Frazee BW, Snoey ER, et al. Ultrasound-guided brachial and basilic vein cannulation in emergency department patients with difficult intravenous access. Ann Emerg Med 1999;34(6):711–4.

12. Schoenfeld E, Shokoohi H, Boniface K. Ultrasound-guided peripheral intravenous access in the emergency department: patient-centered survey. West J Emerg Med 2011;12(4):475–7.

13. Joing S, Strote S, Caroon L, et al. Ultrasound-guided peripheral IV placement. N Engl J Med 2012;366(25):e38.

14. Blaivas M, Brannam L, Fernandez E. Short-axis versus long-axis approaches for teaching ultrasound-guided vascular access on a new inanimate model. Acad Emerg Med 2008;10(12):1307–11.

15. Mahler SA, Wang H, Lester C, et al. Ultrasound-guided peripheral intravenous access in the emergency department using a modified Seldinger technique. J Emerg Med 2010;39(3):325–9.

16. Shokoohi H, Boniface K. Ultrasound-guided peripheral intravenous access program is associated with a marked reduction in central venous catheter use in non-critically ill emergency department patients. Ann Emerg Med 2012;62(2):198–203.

17. Chinnock B, Thornton S, Hendey GW. Predictors of success in nurse-performed ultrasound-guided cannulation. J Emerg Med 2007;33(4):401–5.

18. Miles G, Salcedo A, Spear D. Implementation of a successful registered nurse peripheral ultrasound-guided intravenous catheter program in an emergency department. J Emerg Nurs 2012;38(4):353–6.

19. Stein J, George B, River G, et al. Ultrasonographically guided peripheral intravenous cannulation in emergency department patients with difficult intravenous access: a randomized trial. Ann Emerg Med 2009;54(1):33–40.

20. Sturges Z, Whilte S, Barton E, et al. Ultrasound-guided peripheral venous access by emergency medical technicians. Ann Emerg Med 2007;50(3):S87–8.

21. Walker E. Piloting a nurse-led ultrasound cannulation scheme. Br J Nurs 2009; 18(14):854–9. Available at: http://www.britishjournalofnursing.com.

22. Rose JS, Norbutas CM. A randomized controlled trial comparing one-operator versus two-operator technique in ultrasound-guided basilic vein cannulation. J Emerg Med 2008;35(4):431–5.

23. Grevstad U, Gregersen P, Rasmussen LS. Intravenous access in the emergency patient. Curr Anaesth Crit Care 2009;20(3):120–7.

24. Panebianco NL, Fredette JM, Szyld D, et al. What you see (sonographically) is what you get: vein and patient characteristics associated with successful ultrasound-guided peripheral intravenous placement in patients with difficult access. Acad Emerg Med 2009;16(12):1298–303.

25. Sandhu NPS, Sidhu DS. Mid-arm approach to basilic and cephalic vein cannulation using ultrasound guidance. Br J Anaesth 2004;93(2):292–4.

26. Aponte H, Acosta S, Rigamonti D, et al. The use of ultrasound for placement of intravenous catheters. AANA J 2007;75(3):212–6. Available at: http://www.aana.com/newsandjournal/pages/aanajournalonline.aspx.

27. Bauman M, Braude D, Crandall C. Ultrasound-guidance vs. standard technique in difficult vascular access patients by ED technicians. Am J Emerg Med 2009; 27(2):135–40.

28. Darvish AH, Shroff SD, Mostofi MB, et al. Single-operator ultrasound-guided IV placement by emergency nurses. J Emerg Med 2011;41(2):211–2.

29. Gregg SC, Murthi SB, Sisley AC, et al. Ultrasound-guided peripheral intravenous access in the intensive care unit. J Crit Care 2010;25(3):514–9.

30. Resnick JR, Cydulka RK, Donato J, et al. Success of ultrasound-guided peripheral intravenous access with skin marking. Acad Emerg Med 2008;15(8): 723–30.

31. White A, Lopez F, Stone P. Developing and sustaining and ultrasound-guided peripheral intravenous access program for emergency nurses. Adv Emerg Nurs J 2010;32(2):173–88.

32. Blaivas M, Lyon M. The effect of ultrasound guidance on the perceived difficulty of emergency nurse-obtained peripheral IV access. J Emerg Med 2006;31(4): 407–10.

33. Oakley E, Wong A-M. Ultrasound-assisted peripheral vascular access in a paediatric ED. Emerg Med Australas 2010;22:166–70.

Heart Failure
Pathophysiology, Diagnosis, Medical Treatment Guidelines, and Nursing Management

Chad Rogers, MSN, RN*, Nathania Bush, DNP, PHCNS-BC[1]

KEYWORDS

- Heart failure • Nursing management of heart failure • Heart failure nursing
- Heart failure pathophysiology • Heart failure therapy

KEY POINTS

- Heart failure (HF) is a chronic, debilitating disease that impairs the ability of the heart to respond to increase demands for cardiac output.
- The incidence and prevalence of HF increase sharply with age and the most common cause of HF is coronary artery disease.
- The American College of Cardiology Foundation/American Heart Association and the New York Heart Association functional classification systems are the most commonly used HF classification systems.
- The main aims of HF medical treatment include alleviating or controlling symptoms and enhancing quality of life.

INTRODUCTION

Heart failure (HF) is a chronic, progressive disease affecting 5.7 million Americans and contributes to nearly 300,000 deaths each year.[1] HF is the leading cause of hospital admissions for individuals older than 65 years and contributes to the rising health care costs in the United States.[2,3] The incidence and prevalence are rising as we face major demographic changes in the United States as our population ages. Today many people who have suffered tissue damage from myocardial infarction (MI) survive only to develop HF.[4] Patients with HF usually require numerous hospitalizations. The most common causes of hospitalization in patients with HF are noncompliance with medication, diet, and activity routines, and failure to report worsening symptoms.[3] Because of the aging population and the convenience of effective treatments to

Disclosure Statement: The authors have nothing to disclose.
Department of Nursing, Morehead State University, 316 West Second Street, Morehead, KY 40351, USA
[1] 358 Doe Valley Drive, Clay City, KY 40312.
* Corresponding author. 6214 Emily Street, Ashland, KY 41102.
E-mail address: c.rogers@moreheadstate.edu

0029-6465/15/$ – see front matter © 2015 Elsevier Inc. All rights reserved.

prolong survival in patients with acute coronary syndromes, the incidence of HF is growing and the number of patients at risk of developing this condition is projected to rise dramatically.[4] Nurses in all settings play a pivotal role in managing and educating patients with HF.

Chronic HF develops because of left ventricular (LV) systolic and/or diastolic dysfunction. HF is the only cardiovascular disease with increasing incidence and prevalence, and it has been projected that the occurrence of HF may soon reach epidemic percentages nationally.[5] With HF, the heart muscle becomes enlarged as it attempts to compensate for inefficiency.[2] Some of the general causes of HF include long-term hypertension, coronary artery disease (CAD), poor lifestyle choices, inactivity, obesity, valve disorders, arrhythmias, and some metabolic disorders.[6,7]

HF is a clinical syndrome characterized by a constellation of signs and symptoms.[8] Although medical treatment is aimed at reversing neurohormone and other pathologic responses to decreased cardiac output, the major focus of treatment is HF symptom reduction. With most patients with HF, medical treatment is only partially effective in relieving symptoms.[8] HF is diagnosed by the presenting symptoms and through diagnostic testing.[6] There is a strong need for complementary and nonpharmacological interventions that could be included in palliative care programs to decrease symptoms in patients with HF. The purpose of this article is to provide the nurse with a greater understanding of the pathophysiology of HF, treatment of HF, and nursing management of HF using evidence-based guidelines.

INCIDENCE AND PREVALENCE

HF is largely a disease of the geriatric population and represents the leading hospital diagnosis in older adults. Both the incidence and the prevalence of HF increase sharply with increasing age such that patients older than 75 face a much larger risk of developing this condition. It is the only cardiovascular disease that is increasing in incidence and prevalence.[9] As age is an important risk factor for HF, the burden of this disease on health care systems in Western societies increases as these populations age. In individuals aged 55 years, 30% will develop HF during their remaining life span; that is, almost 1 of 3 individuals. HF continues to be a fatal disease, despite advances in treatment, with only 35% surviving 5 years after the first diagnosis. Prevention of the development of HF in high-risk patients is therefore essential.[9]

It has been estimated that there are currently 5.7 million people in the United States with HF, and these numbers are increasing because of the aging of the global population and the ability of increasing numbers of individuals to survive to an age when HF is likely to become a problem.[2,9] Furthermore, the availability of improved medical technologies has supported more effective treatment of acute coronary syndromes and has conferred better survival rates in patients after myocardial infarction (MI), which is the most powerful predictor of LV systolic dysfunction and risk of HF. As a result, the absolute number of individuals living with compromised cardiac function and clinical HF is expected to rise dramatically over the next few decades.[4]

HF affects more men than women, and its prevalence greatly increases with advancing age.[10] Studies estimate the overall prevalence of HF in the population to be approximately 2% to 3%. From self-reported data obtained by the National Health and Nutrition Examination Survey, the prevalence in the United States was 2.6% in 2006. Studies with validated diagnoses of HF include cohort studies, such as the Rochester Epidemiologic Project in Olmsted County, MN, where the prevalence of HF was found to be 2.2%. Here, prevalence increased with age, reaching 8.4% in those aged 75 years or older compared with 0.7% in those 45 to 54 years of age.

The Rotterdam cohort showed similar trends, with an HF prevalence of 1% in those aged 55 to 64 years, compared with more than 10% in those 85 years or older.[5,10]

In the United States, the incidence of HF generally ranges from 2 to 5 per 1000 person-years, depending on the cohort studied. Like HF prevalence, incidence is greater in men and the elderly. In the Framingham Heart Study, the incidence for HF was 5.64 and 3.27 per 1000 person-years in men and women, respectively, whereas in the Olmsted cohort, comparable rates were 3.78 and 2.89 per 1000 person-years, respectively. At the age of 40 years, the lifetime risk of developing HF is 1 in 5. In older groups, incidence is higher. Based on the Framingham cohort, the incidence of HF is almost 10 per 1000 person-years in those older than 65 years. In HF, which included only those 65 years and older, the estimated incidence was 19.3 per 1000 person-years.[10]

IMPACT

It is estimated that one-fourth of Medicare patients with HF are readmitted within 30 days.[8] HF remains the most common medical reason for inpatient hospitalization in adults older than 65 and reducing the rate of hospital admission in the patient population has become a national priority (US Department of Health and Human Services). Public reporting of hospital 30-day readmission rates and pending changes in US health care reimbursement mechanisms, while controversial, are driving a renewed interest in the development of evidence-based strategies to reduce avoidable readmissions in patients with HF.[5]

The cost relating to HF may be difficult to determine when taking into account diagnosis, treatment, hospital stays, pharmacology, and loss of income. Chronic illness consumes 82% of the health care dollars in the United States.[9] There are an estimated 400,000 to 700,000 new cases of HF reported annually. HF is a major cause of morbidity and mortality in the United States. It is estimated that HF direct and indirect costs in the United States is more than $39 billion annually, and that is expected to increase dramatically in the upcoming years due to demographic changes.[11] In the commercially insured, Medicare, and Medicaid populations, the single largest health expenditure is inpatient utilization (nearly 33% in 2005) with 13.3% of all emergency department visits associated with a hospital admission. The average cost associated with an HF hospitalization is $10,000. Although approximately 14% of Medicare beneficiaries have HF, they account for 43% of Medicare spending.[12]

The prognosis of patients with HF is poor, with 1 in 5 patients dying within 1 year of diagnosis and half within 5 years of diagnosis.[5] It has been difficult to pinpoint the exact reasons for the high rate of HF readmissions. Some areas that have been identified include poor communication, insufficient medication reconciliation across settings, ineffective education, patient noncompliance, and ineffective discharge instructions.[9]

In 2010, the Centers for Medicare and Medicaid Services began to penalize hospitals financially for above-median rates of all-cause readmission within 30 days of discharge for patients with HF. As a result, providers and hospitals now have financial incentives to use effective solutions to the growing challenge of HF management across the continuum of care.[9] This health care reform provision will drastically change the accountability of hospitals for patients' outcomes. Many hospitals have implemented disease management programs to manage these new expectations. Disease management programs have helped patients with chronic illnesses like HF achieve optimal health and control costs. These programs use evidence-based practice protocols, self-help, and patient education and empowerment.[9]

HF touches nearly every important aspect of daily life and patients are encouraged to take responsibility for their day-to-day disease management. Unfortunately, many patients with HF fail to adhere to the complex daily routines.[8] Patients also face many emotional and social difficulties in addition to the complex medical issues.[8] HF knowledge is of critical importance to the nursing professional because it is one of the most common causes of in-hospital mortality for patients with cardiac conditions. The frequency of HF is rising to an alarming rate nationally because of the increasing elderly population. Therefore, the need for education and understanding of the problem is essential for nursing to combat the rising numbers of HF victims.

RISK FACTORS

There are many risk factors for the development of HF. Hypertension may be the single most important modifiable risk factor.[9] The risk of developing HF, because of hypertension, rises as blood pressure levels increase, as the patient ages, and because of prolonged hypertension.[9] Long-term treatment of hypertension can decrease this risk by approximately 50%.[9] **Table 1** displays the causes and symptoms associated with acute and chronic HF.

Diabetes mellitus (DM) and metabolic syndrome are also risk factors for HF.[8,9] Left untreated, these conditions lead to atherosclerosis, CAD, myocardial ischemia, thrombosis, or MI, among other cardiac abnormalities. Patients with DM and metabolic syndrome are more likely to develop HF due to alterations in processing of lipids within the body, high blood glucose levels, and high insulin levels.[8,9] Ischemia associated with these conditions leads to loss of muscle, potential remodeling of the ventricle, ventricular dilation, and ultimately HF.[9]

Cardiomyopathy is a risk factor for HF as well as a potential result of HF.[5,9] Dilated cardiomyopathy (DCM) is commonly associated with HF.[5,9] The prognosis for the patient with HF and DCM is poor, with only a 50% 5-year survival rate. There are several causes of DCM, including obesity, diabetes, thyroid disease, toxins, and tachycardia.[9]

There are several others risk factors for HF. Some diabetic medications have been associated with HF. In particular, rosiglitazone and pioglitazone have been found to increase the risk of HF.[10] Other risk factors include sleep apnea, heart valve disease, congenital heart defects, irregular heart rhythms, obesity, and tobacco use.[10] Tobacco smoking is a major risk factor for HF and smokers should be strongly encouraged to quit.[9]

These are independent risk factors for HF. Yet, these risk factors are also understood to be complementary. When multiple risk factors are present, the overall risk for HF increases. These risk factors should be addressed on an individual basis and, when applicable, on an overall basis.

Table 1
Causes and symptoms/signs of acute and chronic heart failure (HF)

	Acute HF	Chronic HF
Causes	Myocardial infarction Acute valvular lesion	Systemic hypertension Myocardial infarction Valvular lesions Cardiomyopathies
Symptoms/Signs	Tachycardia Hypotension Dyspnea Pulmonary edema Systemic edema	Exertional dyspnea Systemic edema Cardiomegaly Fatigue Orthopnea

From Battista E. Crash course: pharmacology. St Louis (MO): Elsevier; 2006; with permission.

PATHOPHYSIOLOGY OF HEART FAILURE AND COMPENSATORY MECHANISMS

HF occurs when the functioning heart is no longer able to meet the needs of the body. HF is characterized by a decrease in cardiac output.[10] The most common causes of HF include CAD, diabetes mellitus, hypertension, obesity, and cardiomyopathy.[5,8–10]

In coronary heart disease, plaques are deposited along the coronary arteries. Over time, these plaques impede or occlude blood flow to the area distal of the deposit. Therefore, the oxygen-rich blood that is needed is no longer present in the myocardium and cardiac oxygen demand surpasses supply.[9,11] This hypoxia can lead to cell injury and death. As cells die, they are not replaced, and other cardiac myocytes must elongate and stretch to compensate. This leads to hypertrophied, poorly functioning myocardial cells.[13] These changes lead to a weakened myocardium with decreased cardiac output that is unable to meet the metabolic demands of the body.[9,11]

Hypertension leads to an increased workload of the heart. Over time, this greater workload can damage and weaken the heart, leading to HF.[11] As the heart continues to work harder to eject blood, it is eventually left unable to meet the metabolic demands of the body. Proper treatment of high blood pressure can prevent LV failure.

In the patient with DM, high blood sugar levels and alterations in lipid metabolism cause damage to the vessels that supply blood to the heart. This damage leads to decreased blood flow, which in turn leads to decreased myocardial function and potential death of myocardial cells.[11,13] As cells die, neighboring cells attempt to compensate by altering their shape and workload, but as a result they function poorly.[9] This leaves the heart unable to meet the metabolic needs of the body.

There are several other physiologic causes of HF. Among these are heart valve disease and arrhythmias.[5] For instance, when the mitral valve does not shut all the way, blood flows backward into the upper heart chamber (atrium) from the lower chamber as it contracts. This decreases the amount of blood that flows to the rest of the body. Thus, the heart may try to pump harder, which may lead to HF.

COMPENSATORY MECHANISMS

When decreased cardiac output (CO) is present and mean arterial pressure is low, there are several compensatory mechanisms that are stimulated.[5,9] In response to decreased CO, the sympathetic nervous system (SNS) is stimulated to release epinephrine and norepinephrine. The release of these 2 catecholamines leads to an increase in peripheral vascular resistance (PVR), heart rate, and contractility. Because of this, the renin-angiotensin-aldosterone system is activated. Renin secretion is stimulated by a decreased blood volume. Renin then promotes the conversion of angiotensin I to angiotensin II, via the angiotensin converting enzyme (ACE). Angiotensin II leads to vasoconstriction and stimulates the secretion of aldosterone[5,9] (**Fig. 1**).

Aldosterone plays several key roles in the HF cascade. Aldosterone promotes the retention of sodium and fluid. Aldosterone also leads to further impaired arterial compliance. This impairment of arterial compliance leads to increased PVR and in turn hypertension.[9] The increased PVR, hypertension, and fluid retention leads to increased preload and afterload, which contributes to pulmonary and vascular congestion. This pulmonary and vascular congestion leads to the set of symptoms that characterize HF. This constant stimulation of the SNS, along with the synergistic effects of the catecholamine release, combined with the fluid overload and decreased compliance associated with HF can lead to ventricular remodeling.[5]

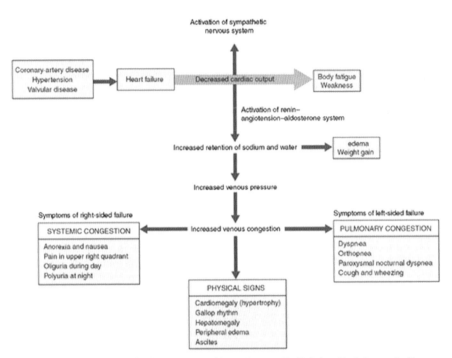

Fig. 1. Chronic HF sympathetic response. (*From* Bryant B, Knights K, Salerno E. Pharmacology for health professionals. St Louis (MO): Elsevier; 2011; with permission.)

CLASSIFICATION

The American College of Cardiology Foundation/American Heart Association (ACCF/AHA) and the New York Heart Association (NYHA) functional classification systems are the most commonly used HF classification systems. One key difference between the 2 is that the ACCF/AHA guidelines recognize both risk factors and structural abnormalities in their classification system, whereas the NYHA scale does not.[9] In the ACCF/AHA classification system (see **Table 1**), once a patient moves into a higher stage the patient remains in that stage and cannot regress. The NYHA scale, on the other hand, classifies HF according to severity of symptoms in those with structural heart disease. The NYHA Functional Classification (**Table 2**) scale is subjective and may change over time (**Table 3**).[9]

Table 2	
American College of Cardiology Foundation/American Heart Association heart failure staging	
Stage A	High risk for heart failure: No structural disease or symptoms of heart failure
Stage B	Structural heart disease: No signs of symptoms of heart failure
Stage C	Structural heart disease: Prior or current symptoms of heart failure
Stage D	Heart failure that is refractory to treatment and requires special intervention

Data from Yancy C, Jessup M, Bozkurt B, et al. ACCF/AHA guideline for the management of heart failure: a report of the American College of Cardiology Foundation/American Heart Association Task Force on Practice Guidelines. J Am Coll Cardiol 2013;62(16):147–239.

Table 3
New York Heart Association functional classification scale

Class I	No limitation of physical activity. Signs and symptoms of heart failure do not present with ordinary activity.
Class II	Slight limitation of physical activity. Comfortable at rest.
Class III	Marked limitation of physical activity. Comfortable at rest, but less than ordinary activity causes symptoms of heart failure.
Class IV	Unable to carry on any physical activity without symptoms of heart failure, or, symptoms of heart failure at rest.

Data from Yancy C, Jessup M, Bozkurt B, et al. ACCF/AHA guideline for the management of heart failure: a report of the American College of Cardiology Foundation/American Heart Association Task Force on Practice Guidelines. J Am Coll Cardiol 2013;62(16):147–239.

HF is further divided into systolic and diastolic dysfunction. Systolic dysfunction is characterized by an ejection fraction (EF) less than 40%.[9] This is also referred to as HF with reduced EF (HFrEF). It is characterized by decreased contractility of the myocardium. Systolic dysfunction results in a thin, dilated heart muscle incapable of maintaining adequate CO. This is the most common type of HF and commonly is the result of damage caused by an MI.[5,9]

Diastolic dysfunction, also known as HF with preserved EF (HFpEF), occurs secondary to loss of elasticity of the myocardial fiber tissue, which leads to decreased filling.[5,9] This is the result of decreased ventricular compliance and impaired ventricular contraction. Eventually, this will lead to an increased workload of the LV and hypertrophy.[5] This hypertrophy of the LV leads to decreased stroke volume, decreased CO, and ultimately symptoms of HF.[5] Diastolic dysfunction is characterized by an EF greater than 50% and concurrent symptoms of HF.[5] This type of HF is most commonly associated with long-standing hypertension.

DIAGNOSIS

Several broad categories can be used to diagnose HF. Diagnosis begins with the history and physical examination (H&P).[9,10,13] There are 3 class I recommendations for the H&P for the patient with HF. A thorough H&P should be performed on each patient suspected of having HF so as to begin to distinguish between cardiac anomalies and conditions that mimic HF, but are not cardiac related.[9] For patients who have been diagnosed with idiopathic DCM, a 3-generation family history should be obtained and vital signs and fluid volume status should be assessed at each patient encounter. Current recommendations for assessing the patient with HF include measuring body mass index (BMI) to monitor weight loss, and blood pressure measurements taken supine and upright; the pulse should be assessed for orthostatic changes and heart tones should be assessed noting the presence or absence of an S3 heart tone.[9] In addition, the presence or absence of jugular vein distention (JVD), size and location of the point of maximal intensity, peripheral edema, and the temperature of the lower extremities should be assessed and recorded at each interaction.[9]

Screening is a class IIa recommendation for the patient with HF. There are 2 main screening tools available for HF.[9] The Seattle Heart Failure Model (SHFM) is an online assessment that can be best used for ambulatory patients with HF.[14,15] The SHFM can provide an accurate estimate of 1-year, 2-year, and 3-year survival rates for the patient with HF. It does so by using clinical, pharmacologic, device, and laboratory characteristics.[9] Patients hospitalized with acutely decompensated HF should have the Acute

Decompensated Heart Failure Registry (ADHERE) model screening tool used.[9] This is an automated measurement tool that identifies patients at high risk for readmission and death. Incorporated into the ADHERE model are 3 variables: systolic blood pressure, blood urea nitrogen (BUN), and serum creatinine.[9]

Diagnostic testing also can be used in diagnosing and assessing HF. Class I recommendations for a patient presenting with HF include a complete blood count, urinalysis, serum electrolytes, BUN, serum creatinine, glucose, fasting lipid levels, liver function tests, and thyroid-stimulating hormone. A 12-lead electrocardiogram should be performed to serve as a baseline comparison.[9] Class IIa recommendations for HF diagnostic examinations include hemochromatosis, human immunodeficiency virus, amyloidosis, and pheochromocytoma testing if it is reasonable to suspect the patient has presented with one of these conditions. B-type natriuretic peptide (BNP) can be used to determine HF presence and progress in both ambulatory and hospitalized patients, as a class I recommendation in both settings. In the ambulatory care setting, a BNP can be used to achieve optimal achievement of guideline-directed medical treatment (GDMT) in clinically normovolemic patients followed in an HF disease management program.[9] Cardiac biomarkers troponin T and I can be measured in the patient with HF and commonly are elevated in patients with HF. Decreasing levels seem to correlate with improvement in HF status.[9]

A chest radiograph is recommended for each patient with HF. This will enable the practitioner to assess heart size and pulmonary congestion. A chest radiograph will also allow the practitioner to glean information about causes of cardiac anomalies that are not related to HF. A 2-dimensional electrocardiogram is also a class I recommendation as a noninvasive diagnostic examination. This test will allow the practitioner to identify abnormalities in ventricular function, size, wall thickness, wall motion, and valve function.[9]

Invasive monitoring also can be performed for the patients with HF. The class I recommendation is for invasive hemodynamic monitoring with a pulmonary artery catheter to influence therapy in patients who have pulmonary distress or evidence of impaired perfusion. As a class IIa recommendation, pulmonary pressure monitoring also can be used in patients who have persistent symptoms despite empiric therapy. Cardiac catheterization is another option that can be used as a class IIb recommendation for patients in whom ischemia contributes to HF.[9]

MEDICAL TREATMENT GUIDELINES

To most consistently treat HF, the ACCF/AHA has developed guidelines for the treatment of HF. Treatments are divided into 3 main categories: medical treatment, device therapy, and surgical management. GDMT is directed primarily by the ACCF/AHA staging system, in which patients are classified as stage A, B, C, or D or by the NYHA classification system in which patients are classified as class I, II, III, or IV.[9]

Patients classified as stage A are at high risk for HF, but are asymptomatic and have no structural disease of the heart. These patients may have uncontrolled hypertension (HTN), atherosclerotic heart disease (AHD), DM, obesity, or metabolic syndrome; may be using cardiotoxic medications; or have a family history of cardiomyopathy.[8,9] The goals of interventions for stage A patients is to prevent vascular disease, CAD, or LV abnormalities. Treatment for the stage A patients is mainly medicinal.[9] Common class I medications for stage A patients with HF include ACE inhibitors (ACEI) or angiotensin receptors blockers (ARBs). These are especially effective in patients with DM, known vascular disease, or HTN.[9,16] Statins are also a medication choice for the stage A patient to control blood lipid levels and prevent atherosclerosis.[9,16]

Stage B patients exhibit structural disease of the heart, but are asymptomatic. These patients have frequently had a previous MI or asymptomatic valvular heart disease. Stage B also includes patients who have LV remodeling. The goals of therapy for the stage B patient are to prevent further HF symptoms and further cardiac remodeling.[9] The recommended medications in stage B include ACEIs or ARBs for the patient with DM, renal insufficiency, or a patient who has had an MI and has reduced EF. Beta blockers (BB) also may be used for the patient who has suffered an MI and has reduced EF.[9,16] Statins should be used in patients who have had an MI to prevent HF. In selected patients, when it is appropriate, device therapy and surgical therapy are also available.[9,16]

Device therapy options for the stage B patient are limited to an implantable cardioverter-defibrillator (ICD). An ICD is a reasonable option for patients who are 30 days or more post MI and have an LVEF of 30% or lower and are currently on GDMT. For patients in stage B who qualify, there is revascularization surgery or valve surgery.[9]

The stage C patient with HF has structural heart disease with previous or current symptoms of HF. There are 2 further subclassifications in stage C HF: HFrEF and HRpEF.[9] The goals for those with HFpEF are to control symptoms, improve health-related quality of life (HRQOL), prevent hospitalization, and prevent mortality. Treatment for HFpEF includes the treatments in stages A and B that are GDMT for comorbidities such as HTN, atrial fibrillation, CAD, and DM. For HFrEF, the goals of treatment are to control symptoms, provide patient education that will improve quality of life and effectiveness of treatment, prevent hospitalization, and prevent mortality.[9] Drugs that are in routine use for patients with HFrEF are diuretics, ACEI, ARBs, BBs, and aldosterone agonists.[9,16] Patients who are classified at stage C, NYHA class II-IV, and have HFrEf with fluid overload and are being treated with an ACE or ARB and a BB should have a loop diuretic added to their treatment regimen.[9,16] For persistently symptomatic African American patients, Hydal-Nirtates should be considered. Patients who are classified at stage C, NYHA class II-IV, and have HFrEf with fluid overload and are being treated with an ACE or ARB and BB with an estimated creatinine clearance of greater than 30 mL and K<5.0, may be treated with an aldosterone agonist.[9,16]

Other medications that may be considered in stage C include hydralazine and isosorbide dinitrate.[9,16] These medications serve to decrease morbidity and mortality, especially among African American patients.[9] Digitalis also can be used in patients with persistent symptoms of HFrEF during GDMT.[9,16] According to the NYHA, a study of patients determined to be class II or III HF showed that the use of digitalis showed no effect on mortality rate, but did moderately decrease hospital readmission rates and combined risk of death rate over 2 to 5 years.[9]

Device therapy and surgery intervention is also available for stage C HF. Cardiac resynchronization therapy, ICD, and revascularization surgery or valvular surgery may be treatment options.[9]

As part of a holistic treatment program, several nonpharmacological interventions should be pursued aggressively. Patient education should be a major component of the treatment for stage C HF.[9,13] The health care team should work with the patient to identify social support systems. Studies have indicated that lack of social support correlates with increased hospital readmission rates.[9] Stage C patients should be instructed to limit sodium intake to 1500 mg per day or less and to have any existing sleep disorders treated and suspected sleep disorders evaluated. BMI should be managed appropriately.[9] Interestingly, patients with HF who have a BMI of 30 to 35 kg/m^2 have lower mortality and readmission rates than those whose BMI is within the normal range (**Fig. 2**). Finally, exercise training is a class I recommendation for the

$$BMI\ (kg/m^2) = \frac{Weight\ (pounds) \times 703}{Height\ (inches)^2}$$

Weight in Pounds

		120	130	140	150	160	170	180	190	200	210	220	230	240	250
	4'6	29	31	34	36	39	41	43	46	48	51	53	56	58	60
	4'8	27	29	31	34	36	38	40	43	45	47	49	52	54	56
	4'10	25	27	29	31	34	36	38	40	42	44	46	48	50	52
	5'0	23	25	27	29	31	33	35	37	39	41	43	45	47	49
	5'2	22	24	26	27	29	31	33	35	37	38	40	42	44	46
Height in Feet and Inches	5'4	21	22	24	26	28	29	31	33	34	36	38	40	41	43
	5'6	19	21	23	24	26	27	29	31	32	34	36	37	39	40
	5'8	18	20	21	23	24	26	27	29	30	32	34	35	37	38
	5'10	17	19	20	22	23	24	26	27	29	30	32	33	35	36
	6'0	16	18	19	20	22	23	24	26	27	28	30	31	33	34
	6'2	15	17	18	19	21	22	23	24	26	27	28	30	31	32
	6'4	15	16	17	18	20	21	22	23	24	26	27	28	29	30
	6'6	14	15	16	17	19	20	21	22	23	24	25	27	28	29
	6'8	13	14	15	17	18	19	20	21	22	23	24	25	26	28

☐ Underweight ▨ Normal weight ☐ Overweight ■ Obese

Fig. 2. BMI. (*From* Lewis S, Dirksen S, Heitkemper M. Medical-surgical nursing: assessment and management of clinical problems. St Louis (MO): Elsevier; 2011.)

stage C patient with HF and cardiac rehabilitation is a class IIa recommendation for the patient with clinically stable HF. For the patient with HF, there are many benefits to an exercise program. Exercise programs have been shown to reduce mortality, improve functional capacity, HRQOL, and reduce hospitalizations.[9]

Stage D HF is refractory HF. This set of patients experience marked symptoms even at rest and have recurrent hospitalizations despite GDMT. The goals of treatment for stage D are to control symptoms, improve HRQOL, reduce hospital readmissions, and establish the patient's end-of-life goals.[9] Although medical treatments that were used during the first 3 stages of HF may continue, several other options are available to patients. Among these are advance care measures, heart transplant, chronic inotropes, pacemaker, palliative care and hospice, and ICD deactivation.[9]

NURSING INTERVENTIONS

The nurses caring for patients with HF are perfectly positioned to improve patient outcomes. There are several tasks the nursing profession can take on that can improve HF outcomes. Armed with an awareness of evidence based practice guidelines that improve outcomes in HF,[13] nurses develop patient education materials for those with HF. Patient education is a key component to improving patient outcomes and this is a role central to nursing.[3,6,8,9,17-19] Assessment is another independent nursing action that can improve patient outcomes.[3,18,20] Nurses also can aid the patient with HF by providing written instructions for patients, implementing telemonitoring programs, and working in quality improvement (QI) programs.

Patient education is a key to successful management of HF. Many topics should be included in effective HF education. The patient with HF should be encouraged to follow a heart-healthy diet[21] that limits sodium. The patient with HF should be made aware that increased sodium in the diet can lead to increased fluid retention, increased edema, fatigue, and shortness of air, which can lead to decreased oxygenation, further cell damage, and worsening HF.[2,8,16,21] Because HF is associated with AHD, the patient with HF should be encouraged to decrease the overall fat content of their diet and increase omega-3 fatty acids.[8,16] Patients with HF should also minimize added sugar, limit refined grains, and ensure they have adequate dietary intake of sodium from foods such as sweet potatoes, greens, bananas, and dried fruits.[16] Finally, the patient with HF should be taught the importance of following fluid restrictions.[3,6,9,13,21] Although the importance of nursing in providing patient education is understood, at least one study[19] indicated that 55% of nurses involved in the study spent 15 minutes or less providing patient education for the patient with HF in relation to medications, diet, and activity. This study seems to indicate that there is room for significant improvement in this area.

Nursing should play a primary role in the ongoing assessment of the patient with HF.[8,21] The assessment of the patient with HF should be based on the patient's need.[21] Fluid status should be assessed regularly.[21] Five key assessments have been identified that indicate alterations in fluid status: orthopnea, peripheral edema, weight gain, the need to increase baseline diuretic dose, and JVD. Additionally, changes in dietary behavior, activity level, food preparation, new or worsening thirst, increases in fluid intake, and adherence to medication regimen should all be assessed at each patient interaction.[21] If the patient is not compliant with the medication regimen, the rationale for this should be carefully explored.[18,21]

Complementary therapies and healing practices have been found to reduce stress, anxiety, and lifestyle patterns known to contribute to cardiovascular disease.[22] Yoga is known to be effective in lowering stress, lessening depression, and increasing physical fitness and may be used as an adjuvant management program for patients with HF. Yoga may help with routine disease management, prevention of fluid retention, and improving the quality of life of patients with HF.[22] Nurses can integrate yoga into HF care by educating patients of the potential benefits.

An initiative that has recently begun to be studied is telemonitoring. Readmission rates do show improved outcomes with the implementation of telemonitoring.[2,21] It has been suggested that most HF readmissions are a result of noncompliance.[20,21] Therefore, patient education and assessments performed via telemonitoring should revolve around diet, exercise, and medication adherence.[9] A telephonic interaction that assesses the patient's weight, exacerbation signs and symptoms, dietary regimen, medication adherence, activities, and social supports can be effective in decreasing complications in patients with HF.[9] This telephonic interaction should stress to patients the importance of compliance to medication regimen, the importance of maintaining their activity level, and the importance of social supports.[9]

Palliative care is another emerging therapy for patients with HF. Palliative care is indicated for patients with incurable conditions in which medical treatment is no longer effective to manage symptoms.[20] Patients in stage D HF could benefit from these services and should be recognized as a terminal condition. The focus of care should shift from mainly aiming to prolong life to relieving symptoms. There is a great need for palliation of physical and emotional suffering throughout the disease process. Communication to address sources of discomfort and to ensure adequate patient understanding of their disease process and prognosis is integral to the care of these patients. Improved use of palliative measures may improve patient comfort and satisfaction with the death and dying process. This is an area of expanding practice, as a considerable number of patients with HF have end-of-life needs that are unrecognized and unmet.[9]

Furthermore, in addition to the previously listed protocols, there are several other items that could implemented in efforts to define nursing's role in addressing HF. Nurses should also be included in QI programs that focus on monitoring adherence,[21] follow HF GDMT models and protocols, and that focus on patients' and patients' families understanding of education received.[21] In addition, at each patient interaction, the nurse should ensure that vital signs are taken and explained.[13] The nurse should also ensure that patients are managing chronic conditions appropriately, managing weight, and staying physically active.[13,19] Nurses should encourage patients to quit smoking, and avoid illicit drugs.[13,19] Nurses should also take part in screening and prevention programs that encourage healthy lifestyles.[13,19]

SUMMARY

HF is a major public health problem that is at an epidemic level. It is expected to increase dramatically in the upcoming years because of demographic changes. HF prevalence and incidence are substantial. It is essential that nurses in all practice settings have a clear understanding of HF and the pathophysiology of HF, and they understand the treatment and management options available so as to be an effective member of the HF care team.

If timely preventive interventions are not implemented in the United States, HF will become the primary contributor to the burden of morbidity, mortality, and health care costs. Readmissions are costly to the health care system and affect quality of life for patients.[23,24] HF requires patients' self-management at home and can be complex, involving many aspects of daily living, which can be challenging.[13,23]

REFERENCES

1. Heart failure fact sheet. Centers for Disease Control and Prevention Web site. 2014. Available at: http://www.cdc.gov/dhdsp/data_statistics/fact_sheets/fs_heart_failure.htm. Accessed December 3, 2013.
2. Smith A. Effect of telemonitoring on re-admission in patients with heart failure. MedSurg Nurs 2013;22(1):39–41.
3. Wheeler E, Plowfield L. Caring for patients with heart failure. Nurs Educ Perspect 2004;25(1):16.
4. Tendera M. Epidemiology, treatment, and guidelines for the treatment of heart failure in Europe. Eur Heart J 2005;7(1):5–9.
5. Fletcher L, Thomas D. Heart failure: understanding the pathophysiology and management. J Am Acad Nurse Pract 2001;13(6):249–57.

6. Sterne P, Grossman S, Migliardi J, et al. Nurses' knowledge of heart failure: implications for decreasing 30-day readmission rates. MedSurg Nurs 2014;23(5): 321–9.
7. Nicholson C. Chronic heart failure—pathophysiology, diagnosis and treatment. Nurs Older People 2014;26(7):29–38.
8. Lennie T, Moser D, Biddle M, et al. Nutrition intervention to decrease symptoms in patients with advanced heart failure. Res Nurs Health 2013;36(1):120–45.
9. Yancy C, Jessup M, Bozkurt B, et al. ACCF/AHA guideline for the management of heart failure: a report of the American College of Cardiology Foundation/American Heart Association Task Force on Practice Guidelines. J Am Coll Cardiol 2013;62(16):147.
10. Bui A, Horwich T, Fonarow G. Epidemiology and risk profile of heart failure. Nat Rev Cardiol 2011;8(3):30–41.
11. Siracuse J, Chaikof E. The pathogenesis of diabetic atherosclerosis. Diabetes and Peripheral Vascular Disease: Diagnosis and Management 2012;158(5): 13–26.
12. Diseases and conditions: heart failure. Mayo Clinic Web site. 1998. Available at: http://www.mayoclinic.org/diseases-conditions/heart-failure/basics/risk-factors/con-20029801. Accessed 2015.
13. What is heart failure? National Institutes of Health Web site. Available at: http://www.nhlbi.nih.gov/health/health-topics/topics/hf#. Accessed March 27, 2014.
14. Levy W, Mozaffian D, Linker D, et al. The Seattle heart failure model. Circulation 2006;113(11):1424–33.
15. Amarasingham R, Moore BJ, Drazner MH, et al. An automated model to identify heart failure patients at risk for 30 day readmission or death using electronic medical record data. Med Care 2010;48(11):981–8.
16. Bostock B. Drug treatments for heart failure. Pract Nurse 2011;41(5):22–6.
17. Richards N. Evidence matters in improving heart failure. Am J Crit Care 2013; 22(4):289–97.
18. Linhares J, Aliti G, Castro R, et al. Prescribing and conducting non-pharmacological management of patients with decompensated heart failure. Rev Lat Am Enfermagem 2010;18(6):1145–51.
19. O'Donovan K. Nursing care of acute and chronic heart failure. World of Irish Nursing 2010;19(1):33–5.
20. Albert N. Fluid management strategies in heart failure. Crit Care Nurse 2012; 32(2):20–33.
21. Boren A, Wakefield B, Gunlock T, et al. Heart failure self-management education: a systematic review of evidence. Int J Evid Based Healthc 2010;7(1):159–68.
22. Kreitzer M, Snyder M. Healing the heart: integrating complementary therapies and healing practices into the care of cardiovascular patients. Prog Cardiovasc Nurs 2002;17(2):73–80.
23. Kubo A, Hung Y, Ritterman J. Yoga for heart failure patients: a feasibility pilot study with a multiethnic population. Int J Yoga Therap 2011;21(3):77–83.
24. Butler J. An overview of chronic heart failure management. Nurs Times 2012; 108(14):16–20.

Index

Note: Page numbers of article titles are in **boldface** type.

http://dx.doi.org/10.1016/S0029-6465(15)00106-1
0029-6465/15/$ – see front matter © 2015 Elsevier Inc. All rights reserved.

United States Postal Service

Statement of Ownership, Management, and Circulation
(All Periodicals Publications Except Requester Publications)

1. Publication Title	2. Publication Number	3. Filing Date
Nursing Clinics of North America	5 9 8 - 0 9 6 0	9/18/15

4. Issue Frequency	5. Number of Issues Published Annually	6. Annual Subscription Price
Mar, Jun, Sep, Dec	4	$150.00

7. Complete Mailing Address of Known Office of Publication (Not printer) (Street, city, county, state, and ZIP+4®)

Elsevier Inc.
360 Park Avenue South
New York, NY 10010-1710

Contact Person
Stephen R. Bushing

Telephone (Include area code)
215-239-3688

8. Complete Mailing Address of Headquarters or General Business Office of Publisher (Not printer)

Elsevier Inc., 360 Park Avenue South, New York, NY 10010-1710

9. Full Names and Complete Mailing Addresses of Publisher, Editor, and Managing Editor (Do not leave blank)

Publisher (Name and complete mailing address)

Linda Belfus, Elsevier Inc., 1600 John F. Kennedy Blvd., Suite 1800, Philadelphia, PA 19103

Editor (Name and complete mailing address)

Kerry Holland, Elsevier Inc., 1600 John F. Kennedy Blvd, Suite 1800, Philadelphia, PA 19103-2899

Managing Editor (Name and complete mailing address)

Adrianne Brigido, Elsevier Inc., 1600 John F. Kennedy Blvd., Suite 1800, Philadelphia, PA 19103-2899

10. Owner (Do not leave blank. If the publication is owned by a corporation, give the name and address of the corporation immediately followed by the names and addresses of all stockholders owning or holding 1 percent or more of the total amount of stock. If not owned by a corporation, give the names and addresses of the individual owners. If owned by a partnership or other unincorporated firm, give its name and address as well as those of each individual owner. If the publication is published by a nonprofit organization, give its name and address.)

Full Name	Complete Mailing Address
Wholly owned subsidiary of	1600 John F. Kennedy Blvd, Ste. 1800
Reed/Elsevier, US holdings	Philadelphia, PA 19103-2899

11. Known Bondholders, Mortgagees, and Other Security Holders Owning or Holding 1 Percent or More of Total Amount of Bonds, Mortgages, or Other Securities. If none, check box ☐ None

Full Name	Complete Mailing Address
N/A	

12. Tax Status (For completion by nonprofit organizations authorized to mail at nonprofit rates) (Check one)
The purpose, function, and nonprofit status of this organization and the exempt status for federal income tax purposes:
☐ Has Not Changed During Preceding 12 Months
☐ Has Changed During Preceding 12 Months (Publisher must submit explanation of change with this statement)

13. Publication Title	14. Issue Date for Circulation Data Below
Nursing Clinics of North America	September 2015

15. Extent and Nature of Circulation		Average No. Copies Each Issue During Preceding 12 Months	No. Copies of Single Issue Published Nearest to Filing Date
a. Total Number of Copies (Net press run)		1283	1292
b. Legitimate Paid and/Or Requested Distribution (By Mail and Outside the Mail)	(1) Mailed Outside-County Paid/Requested Mail Subscriptions stated on PS Form 3541. (Include paid distribution above nominal rate, advertiser's proof copies and exchange copies)	766	643
	(2) Mailed In-County Paid/Requested Mail Subscriptions stated on PS Form 3541. (Include paid distribution above nominal rate, advertiser's proof copies and exchange copies)		
	(3) Paid Distribution Outside the Mails Including Sales Through Dealers And Carriers, Street Vendors, Counter Sales, and Other Paid Distribution Outside USPS®	223	248
	(4) Paid Distribution by Other Classes of Mail Through the USPS (e.g. First-Class Mail®)		
c. Total Paid and or Requested Circulation (Sum of 15b (1), (2), (3), and (4))		989	891
d. Free or Nominal Rate Distribution (By Mail and Outside the Mail)	(1) Free or Nominal Rate Outside-County Copies included on PS Form 3541	22	11
	(2) Free or Nominal Rate In-County Copies included on PS Form 3541		
	(3) Free or Nominal Rate Copies mailed at Other classes Through the USPS (e.g. First-Class Mail®)		
	(4) Free or Nominal Rate Distribution Outside the Mail (Carriers or Other means)	22	11
e. Total Nonrequested Distribution (Sum of 15d (1), (2), (3) and (4))		22	11
f. Total Distribution (Sum of 15c and 15e)		1011	902
g. Copies not Distributed (See instructions to publishers #4 (page #3))		272	390
h. Total (Sum of 15f and g)		1283	1292
i. Percent Paid and/or Requested Circulation (15c divided by 15f times 100)		97.82%	98.78%

* If you are claiming electronic copies go to line 16 on page 3. If you are not claiming Electronic copies, skip to line 17 on page 3

16. Electronic Copy Circulation	Average No. Copies Each Issue During Preceding 12 Months	No. Copies of Single Issue Published Nearest to Filing Date
a. Paid Electronic Copies		
b. Total paid Print Copies (Line 15c) + Paid Electronic copies (Line 16a)		
c. Total Print Distribution (Line 15f) + Paid Electronic Copies (Line 16a)		
d. Percent Paid (Both Print & Electronic copies) (16b divided by 16c X 100)		

☐ I certify that 50% of all my distributed copies (electronic and print) are paid above a nominal price

17. Publication of Statement of Ownership
If the publication is a general publication, publication of this statement is required. Will be printed in the __December 2015__ issue of this publication.

18. Signature and Title of Editor, Publisher, Business Manager, or Owner

Stephen R. Bushing

Stephen R. Bushing – Inventory Distribution Coordinator

Date
September 18, 2015

I certify that all information furnished on this form is true and complete. I understand that anyone who furnishes false or misleading information on this form or who omits material or information requested on the form may be subject to criminal sanctions (including fines and imprisonment) and/or civil sanctions (including civil penalties).

PS Form 3526, July 2014 [Page 1 of 3 (Instructions Page 3)] PSN 7530-01-000-9931 PRIVACY NOTICE: See our Privacy policy in www.usps.com

PS Form 3526, July 2014 (Page 3 of 3)

Moving?

Make sure your subscription moves with you!

To notify us of your new address, find your **Clinics Account Number** (located on your mailing label above your name), and contact customer service at:

Email: journalscustomerservice-usa@elsevier.com

800-654-2452 (subscribers in the U.S. & Canada)
314-447-8871 (subscribers outside of the U.S. & Canada)

Fax number: 314-447-8029

Elsevier Health Sciences Division
Subscription Customer Service
3251 Riverport Lane
Maryland Heights, MO 63043

*To ensure uninterrupted delivery of your subscription, please notify us at least 4 weeks in advance of move.

ELSEVIER